The Proletariat Discourse

In this book, Chyatat Supachalasai offers a reinterpretation of Marx's concept of the proletariat through a Lacanian lens, drawing on the works of Karl Marx and Jacques Lacan.

Building on the intellectual connection between Marx and Lacan, Supachalasai proposes "proletariat discourse", which arises from a re-reading of Marx's proletariat through Lacanian psychoanalysis, drawing on key concepts such as the hysteric, alienation, enjoyment, anxiety, and trauma. Supachalasai argues that Lacan's notion of capitalist discourse, developed in the 1970s, reveals an inherent "non-relationship" aspect within this discourse, indicating the position of proletariat discourse. This proletariat discourse encapsulates three essential components. First, it establishes an agreement and disagreement between Marxist political theory and Lacanian psychoanalysis. Second, it posits that Marx's understanding of the proletariat can be redefined and comprehended through a Lacanian psychoanalytic framework. Lastly, while portraying Marx's proletariat as a subject of resistance to capitalism, this discussion connects with Lacan's goal of seeking an "exit from capitalism". However, from a Lacanian perspective, this connection also highlights the limitations inherent in Marx's concept of the proletariat.

The Proletariat Discourse will be of great interest to scholars and readers interested in Lacanian-Marxist partnership, psychoanalysis, political thought, Lacanian studies, and critical theory.

Chyatat Supachalasai is an Associate Professor at the Faculty of Political Science, Ramkhamhaeng University in Bangkok, Thailand. Supachalasai teaches subjects related to political theory, ethics, political philosophy, and international politics. He has authored several books in Thai, delving into the realms of Lacanian psychoanalysis, Poststructuralism, Marxism, and Speculative Realism. His published articles in English examine the theoretical connection between Lacanian psychoanalysis, subjectivity, and political resistance, as well as address contemporary issues in Thai politics. His current research interests include Lacanian psychoanalysis, Marxist theory, contemporary political thought, and trauma theory.

Psychoanalytic Political Theory

Edited by Matthew H. Bowker
University at Buffalo and
David W. McIvor
Colorado State University

Psychoanalytic Political Theory provides a publishing space for the highest quality scholarship at the intersection of psychoanalysis and normative political theory. It offers a forum for texts that deepen our understanding of the complex relationships between the world of politics and the world of the psyche.

Recently Published Books

6. **Winnicott and Labor's Eclipse of Life**
   Work is Where We Start From
   Nathan Gerard

7. **Rethinking Property**
   Drive Theory, Fanon, and Environmental Philosophy
   Elliott Schwebach

8. **Powers of Abjection**
   Politics and Lacanian Ontology
   Ricardo Laleff Ilieff

9. **José Luis Villacañas and Political Theory in the 21st Century**
   Political Theology, Empire, Republic, Populism and Beyond
   Edited by Nicol A. Barria-Asenjo

10. **The Proletariat Discourse**
    Rethinking Marx in Lacanian Psychoanalysis
    Chyatat Supachalasai

For more information about this series, please visit: www.routledge.com/PsychoanalyticPolitical-Theory/book-series/PPT

The Proletariat Discourse

Rethinking Marx in Lacanian Psychoanalysis

Chyatat Supachalasai

Routledge
Taylor & Francis Group
NEW YORK AND LONDON

First published 2027
by Routledge
605 Third Avenue, New York, NY 10158

and by Routledge
4 Park Square, Milton Park, Abingdon, Oxon, OX14 4RN

Routledge is an imprint of the Taylor & Francis Group, an informa business

ISBN: 978-1-041-11001-9 (hbk)
ISBN: 978-1-041-11002-6 (pbk)
ISBN: 978-1-003-65778-1 (ebk)

DOI: 10.4324/9781003657781

Typeset in Times New Roman
by Apex CoVantage, LLC

Contents

Figures

Preface

In light of global protest movements against oppressive governments across various countries, highlighting the widespread discontent with economic and social inequalities underpinned by capitalism and neoliberal ideology, this book aims to reinterpret Karl Marx's concept of the proletariat through the lens of Lacanian psychoanalysis. This psychoanalytic approach, developed by Jacques Lacan, a prominent French thinker, is noteworthy for its dialectical perspective on philosophy and psychoanalysis. I believe that Lacan, particularly in his later works, shows an interest in Marx's notion of the proletariat. From the 1970s until his passing, Lacan provided critical reflections that revealed both affinities and disparities between his ideas and Marx's concepts regarding the proletariat. However, he never fully articulated a discourse on the proletariat in addition to his existing five discourses: master, university, hysteric, analyst, and capitalist. This gap is therefore what I aim to address in this book, leading to the development of "the proletariat discourse".

Lacanian psychoanalysis represents a philosophical and psychoanalytic inquiry into the subjects and objects developed by Lacan. This approach to psychoanalysis is flexible; therefore, it is necessary to engage with Lacan's teachings and original texts while addressing a gap and the absent essence of thought already embodied in the text. In other words, returning to Lacan's original works – to appreciate his insights and intentions – is essential. However, Lacanian scholars can also engage constructively with other thinkers, such as Marx. This collaborative engagement allows for a deeper understanding and offers avenues to enrich Marx's original ideas. As a result, Lacanian psychoanalysis is believed to have the capacity to expand its boundaries in a limitless horizon, suggesting that it should not be restricted to a particular area of knowledge or ideology. In this regard, I would like to outline four essential approaches in which Lacanian psychoanalysis can be utilized in fields of study beyond psychology and clinical practice, primarily drawing upon insights gained from my previous academic journey.

First, Lacanian psychoanalysis can be studied through a poststructuralist lens, with the goal of distinguishing Lacan from other structuralist thinkers, particularly Marx. This distinction allows for a clearer demarcation of Lacan's post-structuralist theories from Marxist philosophies. When I was an undergraduate student at the Faculty of Political Science at Chulalongkorn University, Bangkok, in 2001, I was first introduced to Marx as one of the prominent Western political thinkers. By 2005, while pursuing my master's degree in postcolonial studies at Goldsmiths College, University of London, I developed an interest in postmodernism, identity politics, and cultural theories. During this time, I was introduced to Lacan through a poststructuralist perspective, alongside other influential French thinkers such as Michel Foucault, Jacques Derrida, Gilles Deleuze, and Jean-François Lyotard. Reflecting on my experiences, I recognized that Lacan's notions of "drive" and "*objet a*" could be connected to Deleuze's concepts of "desiring-machines" and "territorialization and deterritorialization". In 2012, I published my first book on Lacan in Thai, aiming to introduce ten key Lacanian concepts through various examples from cultural productions, such as art and film, to make Lacan's ideas more accessible to the Thai academic community.

The second approach is the provincialization of Lacan, which involves relocating Lacanian theory from Western to non-Western contexts, and, essentially, this can be illustrated as Lacan in the Global South. In this framework, Lacanian psychoanalysis serves as a comprehensive tool for critically examining subjectivities, enjoyment, and desire in relation to political crises, violence, justice, anti-autocracy, and democratic transitions in non-Western countries. My understanding of this approach became particularly clear between 2013 and 2017 while I was a PhD candidate in the Department of International Politics at Aberystwyth University. Under the supervision of Professor Jenny Edkins and Dr. Brieg Powel, I was inspired to explore Lacanian psychoanalysis and radical democracy, particularly in the context of Left populism, and the Lacanian Left of Ernesto Laclau and Chantal Mouffe. Consequently, I integrated the valuable insights of Lacan, Laclau, and Slavoj Žižek to develop an interdisciplinary framework with memory and trauma studies, which culminated in the theory of the politics of survivors presented in my PhD thesis in 2017, where I proposed the theory of politics of survivors, supported by case studies from Vietnam, Cambodia, Myanmar, and Thailand. At the time, I also developed a keen interest in examining the implications of Lacanian psychoanalysis in Thai politics. My aim was to propose that a structuralist polarization is sustained not only by ideological difference but also by indicating a cause of a deprivation of enjoyment. This deprivation of enjoyment is part and parcel of the craft of fantasy objectively sustained by different political groups, until this leads to the failure to recognize the traumatized Real – a national collective trauma in which culprits are exempt from punishments.

The third approach is a Lacanian-Marxist framework that integrates Lacanian psychoanalysis to enhance Marxist ideology. This method utilizes Lacanian psychoanalysis to enhance a Marxist political project, aiming to integrate it into an emancipatory agenda. The concept of surplus-enjoyment is particularly valuable, as it offers a new critical lens to examine capitalism without relying on traditional Marxist concepts such as base and superstructure or labor exploitation. I assume this approach could be described as Lacan and Marx as inventors of the symptom of capitalism, merging the insights of both thinkers. Between 2018 and 2023, I was enthusiastic about publishing several academic articles to support this relationship between Lacan and Marx. This is evident in my previous work on the politics of accelerationism and Lacan's concept of the subject as an agent of resistance. It is important to note that this perspective on the connection between Lacan and Marx shares some similarities with, but differs significantly from, the Lacanian Left. I advocate for this way of thinking because it emphasizes the theoretical parallels between Lacan and Marx, aiming to promote a universal emancipatory politics that seeks to challenge capitalism.

The fourth approach I want to emphasize in this book is my current endeavor, which I refer to as Lacan as an inventor of a symptom for Marx: Lacan with and beyond Marx. This goes beyond simply using Lacanian psychoanalysis to support Marxist ideology and the politics of emancipation, as in the third approach. Instead, it aims to utilize psychoanalysis to identify the gaps and limitations within Marxism itself, revealing the unconscious elements of thought present in Marxist theory concerning the proletariat. I recognize the importance of this approach thanks to the English version of Lacan's Seminar XVI, entitled "From the Other to the other", which was released in 2024. Additionally, I have discovered through various works that contextualize Lacan within the original French setting – unlike the Anglo-American academia I am familiar with – that he is hesitant to align his psychoanalysis with Marxism and leftist ideologies. Lacan seems to develop an ambivalent stance toward Marxism, acknowledging both agreements and disagreements. Therefore, it is fair to interpret Lacan's work without merely using it to support Marxism or Old Left ideology. This is especially crucial as there is a risk of Lacanian psychoanalysis being instrumentalized by contemporary youth extremists and activists. Instead, it is more productive to engage with Lacan's psychoanalysis in an academic, creative, and critical dialogue with Marxism, helping especially young students to better understand the foundations of Lacanian thought.

Remarkably, this book represents the fourth approach. As I discuss and reinterpret Marx's notion of the proletariat – the revolutionary agency in Marxism – from a Lacanian perspective, my goal is to strike a balance between the affinities and disparities between Lacan and Marx. I hope that by using Lacanian psychoanalysis to highlight certain limitations in Marx's analysis of the proletariat, I can avoid the possibility of exploiting psychoanalysis to inadvertently uphold traditional leftist ideology. I believe Lacanian psychoanalysis can benefit Marxism by creatively offering alternative insights rather than endorsing Marxist ideology.

Acknowledgments

I would like to express my sincere gratitude to the Psychoanalytic Political Theory book series for providing a space for this monograph. I am especially thankful to the series editors, Professor Matthew H. Bowker and Professor David W. McIvor, for recognizing the value of my work and for their careful guidance and constructive feedback, which significantly helped strengthen the manuscript. I am also grateful to the generous assistance and thoughtful advice from Natalja Mortensen and Charlotte Christie throughout the publishing process. I also appreciate the professionalism of the broader publishing team, which made the experience of publishing my first book internationally both meaningful and rewarding.

My appreciation also goes to two anonymous reviewers who provided helpful feedback and constructive criticism during the initial stage of the project. Their insights clarified several arguments and prompted me to consider perspectives that I might have otherwise overlooked. Their suggestions were invaluable in shaping the early direction of this work.

Furthermore, I would like to extend my gratitude to Professor Soravis Jayanama, Associate Professor Dr. Suphachai Suphaphol, Associate Professor Dr. Kengkij Kitirianglarp, and Associate Professor Dr. Watcharabon Buddharaksa. They took the time to read and provide feedback on the first draft of this work in its original Thai version. Although the book has significantly evolved since that early draft, many of their comments were crucial in clarifying and strengthening the arguments presented in this book.

I am also grateful to my university for supporting this project. In particular, I would like to thank the Faculty of Political Science at Ramkhamhaeng University for fostering an open and encouraging academic environment. This has provided me with the intellectual freedom to pursue the type of scholarship I value. Many ideas for this book arose from conversations and discussions with colleagues, both in formal seminars and in informal exchanges within this academic community.

This book would not have been possible without the guidance and support of many lecturers and mentors who helped shape my intellectual foundations in political science, psychoanalysis, philosophy, and political theory. I am deeply grateful to my PhD supervisors, Professor Jenny Edkins and Dr. Brieg Powel, for their mentorship. I would also like to thank Professor Andreja Zevnik for encouraging me to further explore the Lacanian notion of hysteric. Their intellectual generosity and encouragement have been instrumental in shaping my Lacanian approach to political theory and scholarly inquiry.

I would also like to express my heartfelt gratitude to Professor Dr. Chaiyan Chaiyaporn and Dr. Choltis Dhirathiti from the Faculty of Political Science at Chulalongkorn University, who first introduced me to the wonderful universe of political philosophy during my undergraduate years. Their intense training was memorable and instilled in me a deep respect for engaging with original texts – an approach that continues to shape my scholarly practice today. I am especially grateful for the trust they placed in me by allowing me to lecture in several of their classes. These experiences were inspiring and strengthened my confidence in the intellectual path I have chosen.

I am also indebted to Professor Thanes Wongyannava, who generously allowed me to sit in on his course in 2004, before I began my MA studies. It was the class that I was first introduced to the works of Jacques Lacan and Slavoj Žižek, an experience that broadened my intellectual horizons immensely.

My heartfelt gratitude also goes to Associate Professor Dr. Decha Tangseefa. His example inspired me to step outside my comfort zone and explore new intellectual and geographical areas. Through his guidance, I learned the importance of interdisciplinary thinking and recognized how essential resilience is in navigating the challenges of academia.

I would like to express my deep gratitude to Professor Soravis Jayanama, who has supported my academic development for more than two decades. He has generously read and provided critical feedback on many of my works on Lacan over the years, and his guidance has been invaluable in shaping my intellectual journey.

Finally, my deepest and sincere gratitude goes to my wife, Tiewtiwa, for her invaluable advice, thoughtful suggestions, and constant encouragement throughout the writing of this book. Her patience, understanding, and unwavering support have been a tremendous source of motivation during this long journey. I would also like to acknowledge our orange cat – Koume – whose quiet companionship and comforting presence brightened many long hours spent at my desk.

This book is the result of thoughtful conversations, mentorship, and collaborative engagement with the communities that have influenced my thinking. Although I have gained significantly from the generosity and insights of those acknowledged here, any remaining shortcomings are solely my responsibility.

1 Introduction

A main thesis: proletariat discourse in philosophy and psychoanalysis

Philosophy: truth and preliminary questions

The primary objective of this book is to introduce and develop a central thesis referred to as "the proletariat discourse". This proletariat discourse engages with a foundational principle of philosophy, seeking the speculation of the truth of the object of study, and, in this case, the proletariat is the object of study. This compels the discourse to refrain from totalizing rather than hypothesizing the truth of the proletariat as a human being that is situated in the existing condition of global capitalism. In other words, the primary concern of the proletariat discourse is to shed light on inquiries regarding the proletariat itself. A philosophical question related to proletariat discourse emerges in the context of capitalism. This question is particularly relevant due to the global spread of neoliberal ideology, which is not characterized by Adam Smith's laissez-faire capitalism based on the principle of free and fair competition driven by the profit motive of private individuals (Schneider, 2026, p. 79). Instead, capitalism, driven by neoliberal ideology, promotes the commodification of all aspects of life, alongside deregulation, financialization, privatization, free market fundamentalism, and the creation of subjectivities that align with capitalist interests (Luth and Potter, 2017, pp. 1–24). This dominant ideology has concurrently led to wealth inequality, increased technological innovation, and surveillance of human behavior to enhance technocapitalist monopolistic power (Suarez-Villa, 2009, pp. 1–7), creating harmful effects for both human and non-human lives, exacerbating geopolitical conflicts, and the expropriation of resources in the least developed countries: this ideology is also bolstered by the rise of far-right ideologies alongside oligarchic regimes. These issues are met with collective resentment as diverse groups united in protest, joined by many proletariats across different countries, leading to the question: what is the intrinsic truth of the proletariat itself? If the role of philosophy is to formulate the right question and to develop a conceptual framework that

DOI: 10.4324/9781003657781-1

relates to a question, then the two preliminary inquiries of this book will be thus: first, what does it mean to be a proletariat in the present? Second, what is the speculative truth of the thesis concerning the proletariat?

Though there are various ways to respond to the two given questions, this book revisits the writings on the proletariat by Karl Marx, a German Kantian communist dialectical materialist philosopher. As a dialectical materialist philosopher, Marx sought to reject Young Hegelian idealism to develop dialectical materialism, which serves as a critique of capitalism. As a Kantian communist, his vision of a communist utopia inadvertently reflects Immanuel Kant's concept of the "thing-in-itself" or the "visionary dream", which exists beyond human perception dominated by capitalism, which can be represented thematically as the "thing-as-it-appears" (Kant, 1998, pp. 410–420). Additionally, Marx's conception of a communist utopia aligns with the philosophical tenet of the Neoplatonic One, which supersedes the existing interrelationship of capital, nation, and state in pursuit of an everlasting transcendental peace (Karatani, 2003, p. i; Karatani, 2014, p. 46). Nonetheless, it is valuable not to abandon the proletariat, as Marx argues that proletariats serve as the agency that connects the present and the future in striving toward this visionary dream (Marx, 1988, 1993, 2004, 2021). It is also important to acknowledge the limitations and inconsistencies between the situation of the proletariat in Marx's time and that of the present day.

Reviving Marx's ideas about the proletariat without considering these contextual and temporal differences would be invalid and largely misguided. Thus, to genuinely investigate the speculative nature of the proletariat, it is crucial to carefully consider four fundamental dimensions of the proletariat discourse: its psyche, existence, subjectivity, and politics. Its significance will be emphasized and reiterated throughout this book. This means that while the texts of Marx and his collaborator Friedrich Engels do provide a distinct political analysis of the proletariat – viewing it as a crucial agent for historical change from capitalism to post-capitalism and communism – some significant issues remain unaddressed. Marx and Engels were not psychoanalysts, and during their time, the science of psychoanalysis did not exist. This lack of conceptual tools limits their ability to fully elaborate on and problematize the proletariat's psyche, existence, subjectivity, and politics. Therefore, addressing speculative truth of the proletariat requires insights from psychoanalysis, as science critically engages with these complex issues. In other words, the current global protests prompt a reconsideration of Marx's views on the proletariat, suggesting that one should also analyze and rethink these Marxist views through a psychoanalytic lens. This approach aims to combine Marx's ideas about the proletariat with key concepts from psychoanalysis, enabling an exploration of the affinities and antinomies between the two fields. The result of this exploration leads to a central thesis regarding the speculative nature of the proletariat itself, which one can refer to as the proletariat discourse. This proposed concept will be connected to the two preliminary questions mentioned earlier.

It is essential to integrate Marx's original insights about the proletariat with key psychoanalytic concepts presented by Jacques Lacan. This book views Lacan as a French self-dialectical philosophical-psychoanalytic thinker. It combines Lacan's psychoanalytic concepts with Marx's political ideas about the proletariat. Unlike other psychoanalysts, such as Sigmund Freud, Carl Jung, and Melanie Klein, Lacan demonstrates a unique interest in Marx's politico-economic concepts, particularly surplus-value, and makes a significant contribution to the development of Marxist thought. Lacan's primary philosophical and psychoanalytic project seeks to use dialectical philosophy to advance the field of psychoanalysis, creating a disruption and fostering internal evolution within his own concepts from the 1950s to the 1970s. This Lacanian approach encourages the subject to psychoanalytically reexamine and philosophically reinterpret their sense of self in relation to issues such as repressed desire, the unconscious, and the drive without object fulfillment, particularly in the context of their interactions with the Other. At this point, Lacan should not be seen simply as a psychiatrist or a postmodern theorist. Moreover, Lacan is refrained from being categorized uniformly within Marxist theory or aligning him with leftist ideology – be it Old or New Left. It is also clear that Lacan does not support right-wing ideology either.

Using the dialectic of Georg W.F. Hegel to deepen his reinterpretation of Freud's psychoanalysis, Lacan's nuanced responses to complex philosophical questions, such as the speculative truth of the subject, are grounded in his unique, dynamic psychoanalytic concepts. Hence, to highlight the unique characteristics of the proletariat from a psychoanalytic perspective, it is essential to rethink Marx's original ideas through the lens of Lacanian psychoanalysis. In particular, the proletariat discourse can also be referred to as the "Lacanian Proletariat", which represents a speculative truth about the proletariat from a Lacanian standpoint. This Lacanian perspective on the proletariat primarily emphasizes an epistemological discrepancy rather than conformity when compared to Marx's original insights. Exploring this Lacanian reinterpretation of Marx can enhance understanding of both the strengths and limitations of Marx's theory of revolution, particularly concerning the possible and limited role of the proletariat as an active agent in the abolition of capitalism.

Psychoanalysis: a Lacanian psychoanalysis

What is Lacanian psychoanalysis, and how has it historically evolved? When does Lacanian psychoanalysis begin to form an ambivalent relationship with Marx's philosophy while also showing interest in Marx's concept of the proletariat? The origins of Lacanian psychoanalysis can be traced back to 1953, the year of Lacan's Seminar I. Prior to this, Lacan was in what can be described as a "crude stage of Lacan" (pre–1949) as a medical practitioner, which was quite distinct from the "early Lacan" phase (1949–1960). During this early period, his work in psychoanalysis was broadly connected not only to the psychiatric community but also to the philosophy and social science audiences. The intellectual history of Lacanian psychoanalysis begins with this early Lacan phase. From this initial phase onward, one of the main characteristics of Lacanian psychoanalysis is its focus on understanding the condition of human beings in relation to the formation of the subject and language. In this context, Lacan shares and moves beyond a viewpoint of Claude Lévi-Strauss by addressing that a human being refers to a subject that is inevitably and fundamentally entangled in the socio-cultural symbolic framework. However, Lacan argues that the subject ontologically is not consistent to a discourse; the subject "escapes his own words" regulated by a discourse, pointing out to the subject as "an interruption of discourse" within the discourse itself (Lacan, 1991b, p. 268). A notable example is Lacan's paper on the "mirror stage", which he presented in 1949. In this work, he began to criticize the prevailing symbolic order endorsed by Lévi-Strauss, likening it to a "Hegelian murder" that shapes the dialectic of the subject (Lacan, 2006c, p. 80). This process compels individuals to conform to the master-signifier, preventing them from being their true selves.

The early Lacan can be viewed as aligning with a structuralist perspective. This is discovered in his assertion that a subject's failure to consistently engage with a symbolic order and its quilting point can result in a psychotic breakdown, as illustrated by Lacan in Seminar III through the case of President Schreber. However, it is essential to clarify that Lacanian psychoanalysis does not solely focus on a subject who forges a smooth relationship with the symbolic framework. Instead, it seeks to uncover the true essence of the subject (Lacan, 1997, pp. 16–28). Lacan describes this true essence as that of a thinking being, particularly highlighted through psychotic language. This language manifests as a non-signified signifier related to the death drive, as noted in Seminar II (Lacan, 1988, pp. 221–234). This unique aspect of the signifier exists outside the reality constructed by the symbolic framework, diverging from Ferdinand de Saussure's affirmative concept of linguistic signification. When the symbolic order is understood psychoanalytically as a delusional fantasy, the subject begins to recognize this framework as both a fantasy and a void of truth. One interpretation of fantasy is that it serves as a veil that the subject wears, performing when relating to others, allowing the symbolic to persist in finitude. Nonetheless, the subject exists in a state of separation – termed "*ex-sistence*" by Lacan – resisting this delusional symbolic confinement by refusing to compromise on their desires. Jacques Alain-Miller (2016) entails Lacan's *ex-sistence* that the subject has to consistently endure with symbolic confinement in order to finally exit from it, even to become "real", which is uncastrated by the symbolic order (p. 20). This resistance is regarded as one of the moral goals of Lacanian psychoanalysis, as noted in Seminar VII (Lacan, 1992, pp. 371–381). Additionally, it is worth mentioning that Lacan rarely discussed the philosophies of Marx and Marxism during his early stages of thought.

In the stage referred to as "mid Lacan" (1960–1968), Lacan continues to focus on the tension that arises for the subject within the symbolic universe. However, his work would have seemed dull and failed to attract philosophical audiences if he had not incorporated key aspects of phenomenology and existentialism. During this period, Lacan draws on elements of thought found in the existentialism of Jean-Paul Sartre and Søren Kierkegaard, as well as the phenomenology of Immanuel Kant, Martin Heidegger, and, critically, Hegel. This engagement allows for an evolution in Lacanian psychoanalysis. A notable example is found in Seminar XIV, where Lacan discusses the enjoyment of the slave as an emblem of the Real, which he describes since Seminar I as something that "resists symbolization absolutely" (Lacan, 1991a, p. 66). The enjoyment on the side of the slave stands in stark contrast to that of the master. The master imposes their enjoyment onto the slave, creating a misunderstanding that the master's enjoyment is actually the slave's own, culminating in a paradoxical logic of fantasy on the side of the slave. For the slave, as a radical subject, it is essential to traverse this fantasy, especially given that the slave's existence is fundamentally different from that of the master (Lacan, 1967, p. 235). Through this relationship, Lacanian psychoanalysis invigorates philosophical inquiries related to the subject, psyche, truth, ontology, existence, and the object of fantasy. Yet, the philosophy of Marx and Marxism is mentioned sporadically during this mid-stage of Lacan.

The political events of May 1968, when French Marxist youths and protesters marched against the national government in Paris, prompted many French thinkers – such as Michel Foucault, Jacques Derrida, Gilles Deleuze, and even Lacan himself – to shift their intellectual perspectives. This period can be identified as the "late Lacan" (1968–1980), which this book refers to as post-1968 Lacan. It represents a time when Marx's critical ideas on capitalism and the proletariat gained more prominence in Lacanian psychoanalysis. A significant example of this shift is Lacan's concept of capitalist discourse, which he introduced to an audience on May 12, 1972, in Milan. In 1973, Lacan (1990, p. 16) introduced the idea that some individuals might "exit" or seek "the way out" of capitalist discourse. This notion inspired and laid the groundwork for developing the proposed proletariat discourse in this book. However, from Lacan's perspective, finding a way out of capitalist discourse is an ethical choice made by certain people. Importantly, this foundational thesis for exiting capitalist discourse does not transform those individuals into saintly figures. As Lacan (1990) states, "the more saints, the more laughter: that's my principle, to wit, the way out of capitalist discourse – which will not constitute progress if it happens only for some" (p. 16). In light of Lacan's warning, proletariat discourse refuses to present a thesis as a means to sainthood. While it may signal a potential historical transition leading to progress, it also allows for space for disagreement and controversy arising from differing perspectives.

During this phase of the late Lacan, Lacan developed nonetheless a complex relationship with Marx and Marxism, one marked by both affinity and opposition, until his death in 1981. In this period, the concept of surplus-value and the idea of the proletariat became increasingly intertwined with Lacan's psychoanalytic theories. In fact, Marx's notion of surplus-value inspired Lacan's invention of the term "surplus-enjoyment", although the two concepts are not identical or easily reconciled. It is important to note that this does not mean Lacan is a Marxist. Lacan was, in fact, critical of Marx and traditional Marxism. Hegelian dialectics is a mode of thinking that still plays a significant role in the late Lacan. This influence is evident in his conceptual frameworks of master and hysteric discourses presented in Seminar XVII, which incorporate Hegel's Master-Slave dialectic (Lacan, 2007b, pp. 11–14). Furthermore, Seminar XXII, which focuses on the Real, Symbolic, and Imaginary (RSI), corresponds with Lacan's interpretation of Hegelian ideas of Synthesis (the subject is a substance of *ex-sistence*), Antithesis (the subject experiencing symbolic castration of desire), and Thesis (the subject's self-perception), respectively (Lacan, 1975, p. 95). This suggests that Lacanian psychoanalysis – across its early, middle, and late phases – has been consistently inspired by Hegelian philosophy, a philosophy introduced to Lacan by Alexandre Kojève in the 1950s (Roudinesco, 2005, p. 103).

Proletariat: the late Lacan inspiration

The concept of proletariat discourse is a thesis drawing inspiration from the late Lacan. In this stage of Lacan's thought, it becomes apparent that Marx's proletariat appears to be Lacan's personal slip of the tongue. The idea of the proletariat, as presented by Marx and Marxism, appears to occupy a lingering presence in Lacan's mind. One contributing factor is the demographic of his late audience, which included French Marxists and Maoists. Lacan occasionally references the term "proletariat" in various seminars and conversations with acquaintances, yet he never elaborates on it psychoanalytically in depth before his death. What the late Lacan hints about the proletariat is that "there is only one social symptom: each individual actually is a proletariat" (Lacan, 1974, p. 187 as cited in Vanheule, 2016, p. 4). In a situation where capitalism is highly exploitative, Lacan suggests that every subject becomes proletarianized because they are unaware of being dispossessed of their own knowledge (Lacan, 1969–1970 as cited in Vanheule, 2016, p. 9). Further elaborating the topic about proletariat still becomes a significant legacy that Lacan leaves for his followers. Rethinking Marx's concept of the proletariat psychoanalytically may bridge a gap in Lacan's personal desire. Consequently, Lacanians have a valuable opportunity to further explore and elevate the psychoanalytic investigation of the proletariat in light of Lacan's absence. Embracing this gap and challenge could yield profound insights and deepen our understanding of this vital subject.

The central thesis of Lacanian psychoanalysis and Marxism regarding the proletariat reveals a commonality when representing a deviation from the master-signifier that governs the meaning of the proletariat. When viewed through the lens of Lacanian psychoanalysis, the concept of the proletariat takes on a different essence compared to traditional definition. In classical economic theory, the proletariat is viewed as a labor force that sells its work for wages. This group is often exploited and regarded as the lowest tier in the economic hierarchy (Dooley, 2005, pp. 162–184). While such definition is not incorrect, it overlooks a psychoanalytic perspective that could enhance a collective general understanding of the term. Throughout this book, by applying Lacanian psychoanalysis to explore the four fundamental dimensions of proletariat discourse, one can redefine the proletariat, moving beyond the conventional notion that serves as master-signifier. This approach corresponds with Marx's radical perspective on the proletariat, as he often uses the term "proletariat" interchangeably with "communist" (Marx, 2007, p. 141). This understanding also supports the establishment of the political regime in which the state is destined toward "*the revolutionary dictatorship of the proletariat*" (Marx, 2021, p. 222: italics original). Certainly, Marx's interpretation of the proletariat also stands in opposition to the master-signifier, which, in this context, refers to classical economic theory. But Lacan critically observes that Marx's understanding of the proletariat often becomes a discourse that effects no change (Lacan, 1974, p. 27). In "La troisième" – one of the crucial works of the late Lacan written in 1974 – it is worth highlighting that "there is no social symptom: each individual is actually a proletariat" (Lacan, 1974, p. 27). In addition, what is also worth considering is that Lacan does not establish a clear connection to Marx. His original insight reveals a social symptom identified by psychoanalysis:

> there has no discourse with which to make a social connection, in other words a semblance. It is this that Marx was working against, was working against in an incredible way. No sooner said than done. What he produces implies that there is nothing to change.
>
> (Lacan, 1974, p. 27)

This means that Marx tends to produce a philosophical-political thinking of the proletariat that forms social connection, but what he produces is ideologically driven and transcendentally unchanged. The highlight of the late Lacan in "La troisième" is that a discourse that forms social connection is impossible, and Marx is the one who works against this rule, insisted by psychoanalysis. Hence, psychoanalysis needs to invent a symptom for Marx's thinking on the proletariat, not just to comply with it. If there is a chance for psychoanalysis to remain a symptom to Marxism, then, "everything depends on whether the Real insists" (Lacan, 1974, p. 27), meaning that Lacan suggests anyone who re-reads

Marx's philosophy, psychoanalytically, to identify and acknowledge the Real – emphasized as a symptom – in Marx's thinking about the proletariat, and only doing this way that psychoanalysis can avoid its death and failure (Lacan, 1974, p. 27).

Consequently, this book, by following the late Lacan's ideas, suggests that Lacan raises doubts about Marx and traditional Marxism concerning the proletariat, not merely aligning himself with them. Furthermore, Marx's understanding of the proletariat as defined by class struggle and class consciousness for the sake of revolutionary dictatorship of the proletariat is not only simplistic, but it can also be seen as another form of a master-signifier tied to the proletariat. Instead of adhering to Marx's and classical economic views, the Lacanian revival and reinterpretation of Marx's proletariat challenges and rejects these master-signifiers. Lacan suggests that the proletariat should begin to engage with the question of identification. This means it is the responsibility of the proletariat to seek and understand their true essence. Lacan is reluctant to define the proletariat merely through class struggle or class consciousness. He states,

> the proletariat are like the Roman plebs – these were very distinguished people. The class struggle perhaps contains this little source of error at the start, that it absolutely doesn't take place at the level of the true dialectic of the master's discourse – it is located on the level of identification.
>
> (Lacan, 2007c, p. 190)

At this point, Lacan suggests that one of the defining characteristics of the proletariat is their self-identification as the Senate and People of Rome (Lacan, 2007c, p. 190), which is assimilated but differs from Marx's class struggle.

If Marx confines the proletariat by linking them to class struggle and class consciousness, this may hinder the proletariat from achieving the level of identification, revitalizing and redefining their speculative truth. It effectively limits their ability to engage in a dialectic against Marxism as the master discourse. Lacan is also concerned with the proletariat as it relates to the function of knowledge (Lacan, 2007a, p. 149). However, the traditional Marxism emphasis on class struggle diminishes this knowledge function concerning the proletariat's speculative truth. While there is a certain affinity between Lacan and Marx, this book, which aims to articulate the proletariat discourse, must also consider the points of antagonism and disparity between Lacan and Marx. In other words, to properly apply Lacanian psychoanalysis in relation to Marxism, it is essential to avoid reinforcing traditional Left Marxist ideology. The proper approach is to identify a point where a Lacanian coordination with Marx and traditional Marxism is feasible, while also acknowledging the ontological tension or the self-inflicted ontological gap within Marx's concept of the proletariat. Ultimately, a Lacanian psychoanalytic intervention can reframe and illuminate Marx's portrayal of the proletariat, presenting it as the uncanniness distinct from Marx's original conception. This leads to the question: how is the discourse of the proletariat, which intertwines Lacanian psychoanalysis and Marxism, produced?

A methodological procedure: producing a Lacanian proletariat discourse

The term "discourse" in the context of proletariat discourse does not refer to a social construction of truth that reflects a power dynamic in the production of knowledge, which is often assumed to be truth and socially propagated to the subject (Foucault, 1980, pp. 109–133). Instead, in relation to Lacan's four discourses (master, university, hysteric, and analytic), the meaning of discourse here draws from Lacan's analytic discourse. Analytic discourse represents a speech act that forms a social bond between the analyst and the analysand. In line with Lacan's analytic discourse, this book develops the term "discourse" not in a Foucaultian context but as a speech act that contributes to the reimagination that attempts to re-represent the speculative truth of Marx's proletariat. This discourse involves exploring the hidden subject of Marx's proletariat, while considering elements such as the hysteric, the unconscious, desire, positive alienation, anxiety, and post-traumatic subjectivity. This exploration serves as a signifier of uncanniness in relation to Marx's original conception of the proletariat and challenges the dominant economic theories that impose a master-signifier upon the proletariat.

To clarify the reasoning behind the term "discourse" employed in this book, it is important to understand that the analysand is assumed to have autonomy. In this context, the transfer of repressed and unconscious desires occurs from the analysand to the analyst, who is expected to minimize countertransference. The analysand's expressions, including hidden desires, are viewed as essential insights that enable the analysand to become the "subject supposed to know" (Lacan, 1999, p. 67). This refers to the recognition that the analysand has hidden desires and symptoms that they are unaware of. The role of the analyst is to signal, inform, and produce discourse regarding the context of the analysand's unconscious and symptoms, a potential or speculative truth. As Lacan notes in Seminar XX, the analyst is meant to interpret and read the subject's unconscious or repressed desires transferred to them (Lacan, 1999, p. 67).

From the book's use of the term "discourse" to the methodological question: How is proletariat discourse produced? How might Lacanian create a discourse about the proletariat? During his lifetime, Lacan did not revisit Marx's works to establish a framework for a proletariat discourse for Lacanian scholars. Nonetheless, there are various adaptable methods for Lacanian scholars to engage with the topic of the proletariat. In this book, the proletariat discourse arises from the integration of Lacan's psychoanalytic concepts and Marx's discussions on the proletariat (Marx, 1988, p. 222, 1993, p. 9, 2004, pp. 49, 20), creating a psychoanalytic reinterpretation of Marx's original ideas about the proletariat.

To begin with Marx, his discussion of the proletariat is extensive and appears throughout many of his works. This book focuses on five key concepts that encapsulate Marx's thesis regarding the proletariat: (1) the specter of communism, (2) commodity fetishism, (3) enjoyment, (4) surplus-value, and (5) dialectical materialism. These five concepts represent Marx's insights into the nature and conditions of the proletariat.

To incorporate Lacanian psychoanalysis into the interpretation of Marx's concept of the proletariat, it is essential to first understand the specific positioning of the proletariat within the discourse. While capitalist discourse functions by exploiting infinite desire and creating a sense of dissatisfaction in individuals, especially consumerist individuals, proletariat discourse can be seen as an unconscious element ingrained within capitalist discourse. Engaging directly with capitalist discourse often highlights the surplus-enjoyment associated with the drive for the profit accumulation of the capitalist subject – the desire of the Other – in stimulating consumers' desire within the realm of consumerism (Bryant, 2008, p. 13). The problem is that critiquing capitalism from this perspective reflects bourgeois enjoyment, signifying a middle-class consumerist subject who enjoys an impossible fulfillment of desire in the realm of market. This approach risks neglecting Marxist analysis of the proletariat and may lead to a depoliticized view toward proletariat's emancipation. In other words, this interpretation of capitalist discourse entirely mutes a thinking position of proletariats, who find the impossibility in the same category of bourgeois enjoyment but are disowned by their products and, ironically, given the inflation and market economy, need to purchase their own products at a miserably high cost. Conversely, if one approaches capitalist discourse from the opposite direction, one will uncover Lacan's insights regarding the proletariat. Understanding this involves delving into the context of the late Lacan, particularly around his formulation of capitalist discourse. It is fascinating to note that the proletariat represents a concept Lacan might have wanted to express within capitalist discourse but chose not to articulate openly. Additionally, Alain Miller's suggestion is significant in that if Lacan were to reconsider these ideas today, his formalization of capitalist discourse might be different from his original insight (Ranzini, 2022).

In addition, developing a discourse on the proletariat requires a psychoanalytic approach to Marx's conception of the proletariat. To achieve this, five Lacanian concepts will be integrated with Marx's five key ideas. The chosen Lacanian concepts – (1) hysteric, (2) alienation, (3) surplus-enjoyment, (4) anxiety, and (5) trauma – will enable a reexamination and reimagining of Marx's understanding of the proletariat. This will give rise to a Lacanian concept named proletariat discourse: the title of this book. This Lacanian proletariat imaginary will orchestrate the four fundamental dimensions of the proletariat, comprised of the proletariat's psyche, existence, subject, and politics. It will highlight both the shared elements and the significant deviations from Marx's original conception of the proletariat.

The four fundamental dimensions of proletariat discourse

A Lacanian engagement with Marx unravels a complex relationship that extends beyond a simple comparison – what might be considered a homology in their critique of capitalism and reflections on the proletariat – between the two thinkers. Lacan suggests that Marx's conceptualization can be viewed as the knowledge of the Other. When this knowledge, such as Marx's understanding of the proletariat, is reexamined through a psychoanalytic lens, it "never reproduces the same, never the same being of knowledge" (Lacan, 1999, p. 97). The knowledge of the Other must confront a sense of lack. There is something new that emerges, one that "does not presume that the Other knows anything about it" (Lacan, 1999, p. 97). This new development occurs at the core of knowledge precisely because the knowledge of the Other named Marx's proletariat is unaware of its own lack until psychoanalysis intervenes to illuminate it.

Reviving Marx while overlooking certain symptoms and gaps in his understanding represents a scholarly movement that seeks to commercialize Marx's ideas in "the age of supermarkets" (Lacan, 1999, p. 98), where scholars must recognize what they are capable of reproducing Marx's knowledge, even through one's existence. In this psychoanalytic context, the attempt to pinpoint a deficiency in Marx's knowledge does not equate Lacanian psychoanalysis directly with Marxism. Lacan introduces the term *commarxe*, which combines the words "commerce" and "Marx" together (Lacan, 1999, p. 97). Lacan asserts that "with Marx's knowledge of politics – which is not nothing – one cannot do '*commarxe*', if you will allow me" (1999, p. 97; italics originals).

Based on Lacan's *commarxe*, a combination of Lacan's psychoanalysis and Marx's knowledge without showing a trail of difference is almost impossible in avoiding a reproduction of Marx's knowledge. This intellectual movement will end up reproducing Lacanian psychoanalysis and Marxism in the arena of commercialization, to impress the public with the dangerous attitude that Lacanian psychoanalysis shares the same horizon with Marxism and Left politics. This theoretical assumption is fascinating, but seemingly unfair to Lacan's original intention. Instead, it is worth encouraging a room not for entire agreement but constructive disagreement between Lacanian psychoanalysis and Marxism, and to simultaneously rescue Marx's conceptualization of proletariat from maintaining the same transcendental status of knowledge. As a result, this can be described through four interconnected points that represent the essential dimensions of proletariat discourse, ensuring that no dimension is considered in isolation from the others.

Psyche

Psyche represents the human soul. However, Lacanian psychoanalysis approaches psychological concepts by moving away from Gestalt psychology: a school of thought that originated in the 1930s. The theory of Gestalt psychology proposes that the mind processes and perceives relationships between subjects and objects, allowing individuals to organize these relationships into a cohesive whole rather than viewing them as separate parts (Koffka, 1935, pp. 3–23). This transcendentalism emphasizes the importance of distinguishing similarities from differences, which aids in human understanding of the world. Gestalt psychology posits that human perception of the self is wholly organized and determined by relationships with surrounding objects (Nevis, 2000, p. 11). It is closely related to holistic perception – such as the person-centered counseling – where the human brain naturally organizes various disjointed experiences into a unified understanding, helping to facilitate the identification of the self in relation to the current social structure (Tolan and Cameron, 2017, pp. 87–98).

In contrast, Lacanian psychoanalysis, in conjunction with Hegelian dialectics, distinguishes itself from Gestalt psychology by moving away from a transcendental aspect of psychological concepts that seemingly lack revolutionary elements. Lacanian psychoanalysis is defined as dynamically dialectical and has evolved conceptually over time, differing from a transcendental approach. This relates to Derek Hook's inquiry about the subject in psychology and Lacanian psychoanalysis. Hook argues that while psychology and psychoanalysis share some common questions and ideas, there are significant differences between the two fields (Hook, 2018, pp. 1–11). Psychology primarily focuses on achieving objectified goals and seeks a temporal structure in which the individual identifies with reality to attain a sense of unity within the self. For instance, when a colonizer encounters the colonized for the first time, the colonized individuals form their subjectivity based on the reality constructed by the colonizer. This process leads to a sense of unity within the self, and, consequently, if this is the case, there will be no movement for decolonization. In contrast, psychoanalysis is dialectical and much more radical. It emphasizes that the subjectivity of the colonized is primarily shaped and influenced by language. However, language cannot serve as a stable foundation for being. In a dialectical sense, the subject must express itself by transcending a predetermined language that limits its subjectivity. This type of subject is connected to an unconscious desire, which can be conveyed through popular culture and various forms of communication. This allows the subject to seek another dimension of desire and break free from such constraints. This is why the decolonized subject, exemplified by great thinkers like Franz Fanon, can be seen as a being that transcends language of the colonizer. Such a radially decolonized subject can be understood as an event that emerges unexpectedly from the interplay between reality, language, and the subject, remaining unaffected by the existing colonial order.

Lacan utilizes Hegelian dialectical methods to significantly reformulate psychological concepts, resulting in a unique advancement that is unprecedented in Gestalt psychology. Lacan argues that "dialectic is in fact immanent; thus, they cannot reflect upon it without latching in panic onto the most simplistic or the most grossly imaginative objectifications" (Lacan, 2006a, p. 309). For a Lacanian, Lacan's reinterpretation of psychological concepts – Gestalt psychology – which he critiques as "imaginative objectifications", facilitates an understanding of the psyche as consisting of internal contradiction and unable to organize in a cohesive whole, and this will lead to a representation of the content of the proletariat's psyche such as hysteric, alienation, enjoyment, anxiety, and trauma, by not relying on Gestalt psychology but on Lacanian psychoanalysis.

To understand the psyche of Marx's proletariat, it is more essential to examine how Lacan applies Hegelian dialectical method, rather than relying on Gestalt psychology, which serves as a guiding principle to unravel the proletariat's psyche. At this point, the psyche of the proletariat is a complex entity that cannot be reduced solely to the class consciousness emphasized by traditional Marxism. This means that, in terms of Marxism's assumption on socio-political objectivity, class consciousness is a fundamental aspect of capitalism, reflecting the historical struggle between different social classes. However, in terms of psychical realm, class consciousness is not sufficient for understanding the psyche of the proletariat. Since consciousness is only one component of the psyche, the complexities of the proletariat's psyche cannot be fully explained by class consciousness alone. From the perspective of proletariat discourse, it is essential to recognize the dialectical characteristic of the proletariat's psyche, by first moving away from Gestalt psychology and adopting a nature of the psyche discovered by Lacan's use of Hegelian method. In addition, the proletariat's psyche does not emerge by instinct or emotion. It is not the human psyche, such as hysteric, anxiety, and trauma, that determines social being; rather, it is social being, particularly capitalism, that shapes and constructs the various aspects of the psyche of the proletariat – like a montage. Again, this goes beyond a simplistic reduction of class consciousness, which overlooks the potential to explore a broader understanding of the ontology of the proletariat's psyche.

Existence

To understand the proletariat's existence in juncture with proletariat's psyche, the proletariat is enacted to inquire and interpret the surrounding being known as capitalism by separating from and eventually changing it. From the perspective of traditional Marxism, there is a relic that the task of old philosophy is an interpretation of the world in various ways, while the new philosophy is on a quest to change it. Nonetheless, it can be argued that the task of philosophy committed by the proletariat is to interpret the world as it is, not in the various ways distracted, to only focus on addressing the problem generated by capitalism, in order to separate from it, and to eventually change it. By the meaning of existence, proletariat discourse aligns with Lacan's neologism *ex-sistence*. *Ex-sistence* is defined as the presence of a being that is substantial only to the extent that it dissociates from something else (Lacan as cited in Fink, 1995, p. 122). In Heidegger's philosophy, existence represents a refusal to be engulfed by the world of living among others. Lacan builds upon Heidegger's ideas by focusing on *ex-sistence*, which is central to the human experience of finding oneself deliberately choosing to be separate from the presence of being-with-others, referred to as "the Other".

According to Lacan, *ex-sistence* refers to the unique place of humanity, where expression and enunciation are tied to distinctive styles. This includes the use of metaphor, metonymy, non-idiomatic speech, poetic language, humor, and even lifestyle choices. The idea is that style represents the essence of an individual – this is why the opening sentence of Lacan's *Écrits* states, "the style is the man himself" (Lacan, 2006b, p. 3). In this context, style embodies *ex-sistence*. By "falling away" from objectivity and the realm of being-with-others, the cause of human desire (*objet a*) emerges. This departure from social connections does not equate to complete disappearance; rather, it is through this transgression of social norms and the Other that an individual maintains their *ex-sistence* through style. Unlike the knowledge derived from the world of being-with-others, which tends to be diminished and rendered meaningless, style represents a person's truth. The dominant societal forces often seek to judge, define, and "castrate" individuals, but it is through style that one reasserts their existence.

The phrase "the style is the man himself" is accompanied by Lacan's warning that "people repeat it without seeing any harm in it, and without worrying about the fact that man is no longer such a certain reference point" (Lacan, 2006b, p. 3). If Marx's concept of the proletariat serves as the primary actor in emancipatory politics, then, in line with Lacan's caution, they should be aware of the uncertainty, hostility, and significant opposition surrounding their existence before they consider distancing themselves from "such a certain reference point". It is essential for the proletariat to be aware of this issue before initiating any political projects aimed at overcoming capitalism.

Subject

The proletariat subject means that the proletariat forms a certain kind of subjectivity in relation to proletariat's *ex-sistence*. First and foremost, the proletariat embodies a struggle against, and a negation of, the unified ego that is shaped primarily by the desire of the Other, or the desire inherent in capitalism. In psychoanalysis, the unity of ego is an illusion. The subject begins to materialize and emerge following its questioning and negating from the ego. The ego is a quilting point, in which consciousness is forged as a result of the intervention of the so-called the desire of the Other, which is defined by Lacan as the intrusion in the process of subjective formation that everyone cannot avoid (Lacan, 2008b, p. 17). Against Anna Freud's emphasis on the unity of ego in favor of a civilizational unidimensional self, Lacan explains that an event where the negation of the unity of the ego is addressed and no longer misidentified does represent the locus of the subject – the *Cogito* – indeed. In addition, Lacanian psychoanalysis aims to diverge from Marxism's characterization of the proletariat as "the class of modern wage-laborers who, having no means of production of their own, are reduced to selling their labor-power in order to live" (Marx and Engels, 2004, p. 21). Instead, it argues that the subject of the proletariat is more closely related to themes of hysteric, alienation, enjoyment, anxiety, and post-traumatic subjectivity. A distinction between I misidentified or confused as the ego and the subject as I identified as *Cogito* reflects a process of "splitting" (*Spaltung*) unavoidable in the subject, whereby humans and their perspectives on the world exist in tension, dialectics, and confusion. This is a primordial classical stage. In other words, this classical stage shows that confusion and tension arise from the disparity between the ego – a foundation of the self that is influenced, for instance, by the reality of capitalism – and the subject, which attempts to negate this foundation, socially constructed by similar forces. And in the next beyond classical stage, Lacan suggests that the subject emerges as a substance following the negation of the ego, which is predetermined to align with the reality shaped by the Other. In Lacan's own words, "Freud's purpose seems to require us to relate it; it is clear that it functions, in fact, to isolate the subject from reality" (Lacan, 2008a, p. 55).

It is worth noting that this process at the beyond classical stage is difficult to succeed. As long as the subject tends to oscillate between the subject feeling confused as an ego influenced by the desire of the Other and the subject striving to become a substantial subject or *Cogito* that endeavors to go beyond the ego, looking for its purity. This oscillation is driven by the unconscious, which operates based on the principle of dialectics, making it difficult for the subject to clearly distinguish between the ego and the subject, and what is inevitable is the ontology of fragmentary subject. Despite such tension in terms of the formation of subject, the Lacanian subject, in confusing with and striving to separate from the ego, in the end, will actively seek another possible desire that lies outside the framework of the desire of the Other. Upon reaching this apex of a non-classical stage that the subject attenuates tension and confusion, the subject still encounters another difficulty and self-disturbance because such desire is mystical in nature: it is not desire of the Other. Instead, it represents an elusive object that is often beyond reach, existing outside conventional perceptions. Sometimes, it may not even have a social existence, yet it serves as the cause of desire. This elusive object is referred to as *objet a*, and connected to a proletariat discourse, a communist world functions as an example of *objet a*. From the perspective of proletariat discourse, the proletariat is caught in a tension between the ego and the subject, as well as between the subject and the *objet a*. This tension extends beyond merely defining proletariat's subject as a social class in relation to production.

Politics

In the realm of the politics of liberation, proletariat discourse aligns with Lacan's "exit capitalist discourse" and Marx's view of the proletariat as a revolutionary force. Finding an alternative to capitalism is essential; one must not shy away from challenging capitalism. This is why Lacanian proletariat discourse partially aligns with scholars engaged in Lacanian-Marxist political projects. But what is the essence of this Lacanian-Marxist political endeavor? This movement developed independently of Lacan's original intentions and represents a body of knowledge shaped primarily by scholars in Europe and the United States. Over time, the influence of integrating Lacanian psychoanalysis with Marxist philosophy has extended to non-Western countries, including Japan, South Korea, Malaysia, Indonesia, Singapore, and Thailand, which is the author's hometown. It is evident that there has been a significant evolution in the history of Lacanian-Marxism and its radical political principles from the past to the present.

In 1989, Lacanian psychoanalysis was integrated into a critique of the fantasy inherent in capitalist ideology, along with proposals for emancipatory potential, while recognizing that class divisions remain universally intact. This history has been prominently shaped by the works of Slavoj Žižek (1989, 1999, 2008, 2025b), a key Slovenian Marxist thinker influenced by Hegel and Lacan, and who once identified himself as a "moderately conservative communist" (Žižek, 2025a, p. 8). According to Žižek (2025a), under a current holographic history of global capitalism, to survive "we need a radical-rearrangement of our entire way of life towards some form of global solidarity and cooperation, but the urgent need to achieve this goal brings new dangers, so we should act with urgency and care" (p. 8). Daniel Tutt entails this debate on solidarity, raising awareness to the politics of proletariat that "from a Marxist perspective, it is not only the proletariat that self-liberates itself, revolutions since the French Revolution up to May 1968 have depended on the building of solidarities across classes" (Tutt, 2022, p. 129).

Žižek's conservative communist stance appears to diverge from the insights of Left populism, also known as radical democracy, as articulated in the work of Ernesto Laclau, a key figure in the Lacanian Left, whose thinking on solidarity remains ambiguous compared with an ontological denial of political consensus, or making society continually impossible. Unlike the political-philosophical project of Lacanian-Marxism, radical democracy's opposition to hegemonic regimes seems hesitant to regard anti-capitalism – from demanding wage increases and work strikes to seeking alternative social conditions to capitalism – as an essentially universal condition for global emancipation. This hesitation leads the Lacanian Left to develop a new understanding of emancipatory politics that is not strictly tied to class analysis. The concept of Left populism, which includes the Lacanian Left, is widely recognized as a voice for democratic politics. Proponents use Lacanian psychoanalysis to move away from what they refer to as old Marxist class essentialism, aiming to "support widening of social struggles characteristic of the present stage of democratic politics" (Laclau and Mouffe, 2001, p. xi).

By postulating a plural form of social and political antagonism as Lacanian hysterical subject and as the Real, performed particularly through democratic identity politics (Stavrakakis, 2007, p. 19) that encompass gender identity, sexuality, racial identity, religious identity, intersectionality, and influence the contemporary paradigm of cultural wokeism, this perspective provides intriguing insights; however, it may ignore the possibility that identity politics can support a hegemonic order of capitalism. An example is rainbow capitalism. The term "rainbow capitalism" refers to a form of capitalism that profits from the LGBTQ movement, while also sustaining the systems of capitalism, advertising, consumerism, and its hegemonic control (Valocchi, 2017, pp. 315–331). In this framework, anti-capitalism, including critiquing consumerist culture, is treated as one option among many, representing just one identity within a network of multiple antagonistic sites. Despite the Lacanian Left's intellectual movement aiming to challenge oppressive hegemonic regimes, both conservative Right populism and progressive Left populism, or Lacanian Left, represent two sides of the same coin. Both are at risk of hindering the potential of anti-capitalism to foster true emancipatory politics.

Since the 2000s, Lacanian-Marxism has aimed to address the underlying material conditions of capitalism and its apocalyptic impact on both human and non-human beings at a global scale. In relation to capitalism and its resulting discontent, this line of thinking emphasizes the importance of critiquing the capitalist system. Universal emancipation remains ideally unattainable without a critical examination of how global capitalism inflicts negative effects on all beings at the planetary level. Global capitalism is sustained by the ideology of Right populism, which aligns itself with an oligarchical regime that promises to guarantee popular happiness – serving as a veil of fantasy. To critique capitalism effectively and identify its root causes, it is necessary to dismantle this veil of fantasy. This approach highlights the importance of recognizing class divisions and class warfare as essential to global emancipation, rather than resorting to lawless counterinsurgency or terrorist attacks, as witnessed after the events of September 11, 2001. The structure of global capitalism creates a stark division between a privileged group that possesses technology and a new means of production, known as digital platform, allowing them to dictate and guide a behavior of a majority of people (Varoufakis, 2023), and a vast proletariat that, while equipped with technology, is deprived of the rights to participate politically and influence the direction of society. The global protests observed demonstrate that the essentialization of class warfare is a significant and urgent issue, rather than a superficial concern.

The economic crisis of 2008 has even made class division increasingly visible and seemingly unchangeable. Although the analysis of class division is often dismissed by proponents of radical democracy as outdated Marxist thinking, this aspect of class analysis remains relevant today and is not absent from a Lacanian-Marxism perspective. While radical democracy attempts to distance itself from traditional Marxism, it positions anti-capitalism as one of many political options in universal politics. This belief in a diverse approach to political emancipation is useful for expanding Marxism's political proposals. However, there is a risk that focusing on political emancipation might divert attention from the critique of capitalism and fail to address the undeniable need for social change that opposes global capitalism. It is essential that anti-capitalism does not become reductive, relegated to just one option among many in radical politics. Critiquing and liberating from capitalism's oppression and exploitation through a psychoanalytic lens is a long-term project that should be prioritized as a central agenda in universal politics (Dean, 2025; Zupančič, 2023; Tutt, 2022).

From 2010 to the present, following significant political events such as the Arab Spring, Occupy Wall Street, and the COVID-19 outbreak, which led to millions being unemployed and an increase in artificial intelligence replacing human labor. In light of these developments, Lacanian-Marxism has begun to recognize the proletariat as a political agency committed to universal emancipation. In response to global protests, some scholars in this emerging field argue that Marx's concept of the proletariat can be explored alongside a Lacanian psychoanalytic framework (Pavón-Cuéllar, 2011, pp. 70–77). In certain literature that combines Lacanian psychoanalysis and Marxism, the proletariat is portrayed as a political agency engaged in the historical transition from capitalism to a post-capitalist stage (Kapoor, 2020). Some scholars discuss Marx's labor psychoanalytically, incorporating key concepts from Lacan, such as enjoyment (Jayanama, 2024; Tomšič, 2019; Jayanama, 2022), alienation (McGowan, 2024), and the subject as the "ticklish subject" (Žižek, 1999), which provides guiding insights into the politics of the proletariat from a Lacanian perspective.

This book aims to create a framework for understanding the politics of the proletariat through a psychoanalytic lens. There are two points to note. First, it moves away from radical democracy and Left Populism, which have often overlooked the needs of the proletariat and shown a reluctance to seek alternatives to capitalism. Some proponents of these Left populist movements appear to benefit from the current capitalist system. Second, while both proletariat discourse and Lacanian-Marxist politics are committed to anti-capitalism and explore theoretical paths toward the abolition of capitalism, Lacanian-Marxist scholars may not fully capture the essence and key characteristics of the proletariat as seen through a Lacanian psychoanalytic lens that reinterprets and rethinks Marx's analysis of the proletariat, making the belief in the proletariat as a revolutionary agency more complex and problematically leading to a lack of proper engagement in revolutionary action because of the proletariat's dialectical psychoanalytic ontology. This observation aims to encourage discussions and dialogues with the Lacanian-Marxist approach and a theory of traditional Marxism. These arguments will be presented in the outline of each chapter of the book as follows:

Chapter 1 examines Lacan's concept of capitalist discourse within the framework of psychoanalysis, connecting it to Marx's analysis of the proletariat and surplus-value. Lacan cautions against a strictly structuralist interpretation, describing capitalist discourse as a sliding signifier that reflects the position of the proletariat. While it is essential for the proletariat to exit capitalist discourse, their self-ontological deficiency may hinder the revolutionary process.

Chapter 2 reinterprets Marx's concept of the specter of communism by examining it through a Lacanian perspective on the so-called hysterical proletariat. The psyche of the hysterical proletariat, described by Lacan as being aphasic, highlights the ruling class's failure to maintain control, which leads to inconsistencies in Marx's vision of communism. Consequently, the proletariat, viewed as hysterical subjects, struggles to imagine an alternative communist world, diverging from Marx's original ideas.

Chapter 3 highlights the connection between Marx's understanding of the proletariat and key concepts like commodity fetishism and alienation. While Marx focuses on the negative aspects of alienation, which align with Lacan's idea of lethal alienation, he overlooks the potentially positive view known as celebrated alienation. This creates a tension between Marx and Lacan, as Marx views the proletariat as a key political agent against capitalism but has limitations in his interpretation of their subjectivity. A Lacanian reinterpretation suggests that the proletariat is rather caught paradoxically between resisting and conforming to capitalism, driven by their unconscious. This dynamic of the unconscious challenges traditional Marxist views on class consciousness. Ultimately, the chapter proposes that the proletariat experiences two forms of alienation, influenced by the conflicting principles of the unconscious.

Chapter 4 focuses on Marx's exploration of enjoyment within capitalism, which reveals that while capitalists pursue excessive and addictive pleasures, the proletariat is largely deprived of enjoyment. For the proletariat to reclaim enjoyment, a radical social transformation is necessary to achieve an egalitarian form of classless enjoyment. This idea relates to enjoyment as a political factor, where enjoyment is divided between the disenfranchised proletariat and the capitalists. The chapter presents an alternative view, arguing based on Lacan's original idea that the proletariat experiences dialectical self-enjoyment through masochism, sadism, and narcissism, which reflects a proletariat's pathological existence in capitalism. However, divine enjoyment, linked to the Lacanian Woman and Antigone, allows proletariat self-enjoyment to resist capitalism through acts of divine violence.

Chapter 5 examines the connection between Marx and Lacan, linking Marx's concept of the proletariat to surplus-value and Lacan's surplus-enjoyment of capitalism. However, it departs from those viewpoints and offers an alternative view that surplus-value reveals two aspects of the proletariat's relationship with anxiety: their conformity to capitalist productivity to alleviate financial and social anxiety, and how aspirations for a world beyond capitalism, like communism, can lead to disappointment and create another form of anxiety. From a psychoanalytic perspective, the proletariat's Psychoanalytic Act can be seen as a *passage à l'acte*, indicating a struggle with social complexities, or as acting-out, which shows a commitment to their desires despite dissatisfaction.

Chapter 6 illustrates that Lacan's concepts of the RSI inform a nuanced theory of trauma, proposing that trauma is a political factor. This framework distinguishes three types of traumas: Imaginary-Trauma, Symbolic-Trauma, and ultimately the Real-Trauma, which is identified as capitalist trauma. Imaginary-Trauma leads the proletariat to form subjectivities based on self-perception, which may contribute to depoliticization through reliance on medical care. In contrast, Real-Trauma, or capitalist trauma, differs from Symbolic-Trauma, where the proletariat articulates symbolic identity politics, focusing on the abolition of gender and racial prejudices but risks neglecting a critique of capitalism. Despite theoretical differences with Marx's dialectical materialism, the three trauma types are interconnected, highlighting complexity in proletariat subjectivity. It is crucial to view the proletariat not just as labor entities but as post-traumatic subjects willing to confront existing social structures and courageous to embrace dangers.

Chapter 7 concludes that Lacanian psychoanalysis offers a nuanced critique of capitalism that aligns with Marxism to some extent, but it diverges in its analysis of the proletariat. It highlights aspects such as hysteric, alienation, enjoyment, anxiety, and trauma, which traditional Marxism often overlooks. This psychoanalytic lens is expected to enhance Marx's revolutionary theory. Rather than viewing Lacanian psychoanalysis as a complete partnership with traditional Marxism or merely as a support tool for the Lacanian Left, it is more useful to see Lacan as introducing a problematic dimension to Marxism, leading to a development of Marxism in return. The chapter concludes with the Lacanian formula for the proletariat discourse.

Reference list

Alain-Miller, J. (2016). 'Ex-sistence', Translated by John Burton Wallace V and Frédéric-Charles Baitinger, *Lacanian Ink*, *48*, Fall, 15–49.

Bryant, L. (2008). 'Žižek's New Universe of Discourse: Politics and the Discourse of the Capitalist', *International Journal of Žižek Studies*, 2, 1–48.

Dean, J. (2025). *Capital's Grave: Neofeudalism and the New Class Struggle*. London and New York: Verso.

Dooley, P. (2005). 'Karl Marx: The Exploitation of Labour', in *The Labour Theory of Value*. London and New York: Routledge.

Fink, B. (1995). *The Lacanian Subject: Between Language and Jouissance*. Princeton and New Jersey: Princeton University Press.

Foucault, M. (1980). 'Truth and Power', in *Power/Knowledge: Selected Interviews and Other Writings 1972–1977*. Translated by Colin Gordon, Leo Marshall, John Mepham, and Kate Soper. New York: Pantheon Books.

Hook, D. (2018). *Six Moments in Lacan: Communication and Identification in Psychology and Psychoanalysis*. London and New York: Routledge.
Jayanama, S. (2022). *Everything You Always Wanted to Know about Global Politics but Were Afraid to Ask Lacan* [in Thai]. Bangkok: Siam Publishing House.
Jayanama, S. (2024). *Cos We are Lacking: The Politics of Enjoyment* [in Thai]. Bangkok: B&B Press.
Kant, I. (1998). *Critique of Pure Reason*. Translated and edited by Paul Guyer and Allen W. Wood. Cambridge: Cambridge University Press.
Kapoor, I. (2020). *Confronting Desire: Psychoanalysis and International Development*. Cornell: Cornell University Press.
Karatani, K. (2003). *Transcritique: On Kant and Marx*. Translated by Sabu Kohso. Cambridge and Massachusetts: MIT Press.
Karatani, K. (2014). *The Structure of World History: From Modes of Production to Modes of Exchange*. Translated by Michael K. Bourdaghs. Durham: Duke University Press.
Koffka, K. (1935). 'Why Psychology?', in *Principles of Gestalt Psychology*. New York: Harcourt, Brace, and Company.
Lacan, J. (1967). 'Wednesday 31 May, 1967', in *The Seminar of Jacques Lacan: Book XIV: The Logic of Phantasy*. Translated by Cormac Gallagher. https://www.lacaninireland.com/web/wp-content/uploads/2010/06/14-Logic-of-Phantasy-Complete.pdf
Lacan, J. (1974). 'La Troisième', Talk at the Congress of Rome. Published in Lettres del'Écolefreudienne,no.16,1975:pp.177–203.TranslatedinEnglishbyYolandeSzczech. Doi: https://www.researchgate.net/publication/307210365_Lacan's_La_Troisieme_English_Translation. Accessed: April 19, 2025.
Lacan, J. (1975). 'Tuesday 18 February, 1975', in *The Seminar of Jacques Lacan: Book XXII: RSI*. Translated by Cormac Gallagher. https://www.lacaninireland.com/web/wp-content/uploads/2010/06/RSI-Complete-With-Diagrams.pdf
Lacan, J. (1988). 'Desire, Life and Death', in *The Seminar of Jacques Lacan Book II: The Ego in Freud's Theory and in the Technique of Psychoanalysis 1954–1955*. Translated by Sylvana Tomaselli. Cambridge: Cambridge University Press.
Lacan, J. (1990). *Jacques Lacan Television: A Challenge to the Psychoanalytic Establishment*. Translated by Jeffrey Mehlman. London and New York: W.W. Norton & Company.
Lacan, J. (1991a). 'Discourse Analysis and Ego Analysis', in *The Seminar of Jacques Lacan Book I: Freud's Paper on Technique 1953–1954*. Translated by John Forrester. London and New York: W.W. Norton & Company.
Lacan, J. (1991b). 'Truth Emerges from the Mistake', in *The Seminar of Jacques Lacan Book I: Freud's Paper on Technique 1953–1954*. Translated by John Forrester. London and New York: W.W. Norton & Company.
Lacan, J. (1997). 'The Meaning of Delusion', in *The Seminar of Jacques Lacan Book III: The Psychoses 1955–1956*. Translated by Russell Grigg. London and New York: W.W. Norton & Company.
Lacan, J. (1999). 'God and Woman's Jouissance', in *The Seminar of Jacques Lacan: Book XX: On Feminine Sexuality: The Limits of Love and Knowledge, 1972–1973*. Translated by Bruce Fink. London and New York: W.W. Norton and Company.
Lacan, J. (2006a). 'Introduction to Jean Hyppolite's Commentary on Freud's "Verneinung"', in *Écrits: The First Complete Edition in English*. Translated by Bruce Fink. London and New York: W.W. Norton & Company.
Lacan, J. (2006b). 'Overture to this Collection', in *Écrits: The First Complete Edition in English*. Translated by Bruce Fink. London and New York: W.W. Norton & Company.
Lacan, J. (2006c). 'The Mirror Stage as Formative of the *I* Function as Revealed in Psychoanalytic Experience', in *Écrits: The First Complete Edition in English*. Translated by Bruce Fink. London and New York: W.W. Norton & Company.

Lacan, J. (2007a). 'Interview on the steps of the Pantheon', in *The Seminar of Jacques Lacan: Book XVII: The Other Side of Psychoanalysis*. Translated by Russell Grigg. London and New York: W.W. Norton and Company.
Lacan, J. (2007b). 'Production of the Four Discourses', in *The Seminar of Jacques Lacan: Book XVII: The Other Side of Psychoanalysis*. Translated by Russell Grigg. London and New York: W.W. Norton and Company.
Lacan, J. (2007c). 'The power of the impossibles', in *The Seminar of Jacques Lacan: Book XVII: The Other Side of Psychoanalysis*. Translated by Russell Grigg. London and New York: W.W. Norton and Company.
Lacan, J. (2008a). '*Das Ding*', in *The Seminar of Jacques Lacan Book VII: The Ethics of Psychoanalysis*. Translated by Dennis Porter. Edited by Jacques-Alain Miller. London and New York: Routledge.
Lacan, J. (2008b). 'Outline of the Seminar', in *The Seminar of Jacques Lacan Book VII: The Ethics of Psychoanalysis*. Translated by Dennis Porter. Edited by Jacques-Alain Miller. London and New York: Routledge.
Laclau, E., and Chantal Mouffe (2001). *Hegemony and Socialist Strategy*. 2nd Edition. London and New York: Verso.
Luth, J., and Martin Potter (2017). *Edges of Identity: The Production of Neoliberal Subjectivities*. Chester: University of Chester Press.
Marx, K. (1988). *Economic and Philosophic Manuscripts of 1844*. New York: Prometheus Book.
Marx, K. (1993). *Grundrisse: Foundations of the Critique of Political Economy*. London: Penguin Classics.
Marx, K. (2007). "The German Ideology': Chapter One, 'Feuerbach', in *Marx Early Political Writings*. 3rd Edition. Edited by Joseph O'Malley. Cambridge: Cambridge University Press.
Marx, K. (2021). 'Critique of the Gotha Programme: Marginal Notes on the Programme of the German Workers' Party', in *Marx Later Political Writings*. 2nd Edition. Edited by Terrell Carver. Cambridge: Cambridge University Press.
Marx. K. (2004). 'Manifesto of the Communist Party', in *The Collector's Library of Essential Thinkers*. London: CRW Publishing Limited.
Marx, K. and Frederick Engels (2004). *The German Ideology Part One*. Edited by C.J. Arthur. New York: International Publishers.
McGowan, T. (2024). *Embracing Alienation: Why We Shouldn't Try to Find Ourselves*. Watkins Media.
Nevis, E. (2000). *Gestalt Therapy: Perspectives and Applications*. London and New York: Routledge.
Pavón-Cuéllar, D. (2011). 'Marx in Lacan: Proletarian Truth in Opposition to Capitalist Psychology, in *Annual Review of Critical Psychology*. pp. 70–77.
Ranzini, O. (2022). *Jacques-Alain Miller: "Lacan Foresaw the Global Domination of Capitalism*. New Lacanian School. https://www.amp-nls.org/nls-messager/jacques-alain-miller-lacan-foresaw-the-global-domination-of-capitalism/: Accessed: January 15, 2025.
Roudinesco, E. (2005). 'The Philosophy School: Alexandre Koyré and Others', in *Jacques Lacan: An Outline of a Life and a History of a System of Thought*. Translated by Barbara Bray. Cambridge and Malden: Polity Press.
Schneider, G. (2026). 'Adam Smith and the Rise of Capitalism: The Era of Laissez-Faire', in *The Evolution of Economic Ideas and Systems: A Pluralist Approach*. Oxon and New York: Routledge.
Stavrakakis, Y. (2007). *The Lacanian Left: Psychoanalysis, Theory, Politics*. Edinburgh: Edinburgh University Press.

Suarez-Villa, L. (2009). *Technocapitalism: A Critical Perspective on Technological Innovation and Corporatism*. Philadelphia: Temple University Press.
Tolan, J. and Rose Cameron. (2017). 'Psychological Contact I – Basic and Cognitive Contact', in *Skills in Person-Centered: Counselling & Psychotherapy*. London: Sage Publications.
Tomšič, S. (2019). *The Labour of Enjoyment: Towards a Critique of Libidinal Economy*. Berlin: August Verlag.
Tutt, D. (2022). *Psychoanalysis and the Politics of the Family: The Crisis of Initiation*. Cham: Palgrave Macmillan.
Valocchi, S. (2017). 'Capitalisms and Gay Identities: Towards a Capitalist Theory of Social Movements', *Social Problems*, 64(2), 315–331.
Vanheule, S. (2016). 'Capitalist Discourse, Subjectivity, and Lacanian Psychoanalysis', *Frontiers in Psychology*, (7), 1–15. doi: https://doi.org/10.3389/fpsyg.2016.01948
Varoufakis, Y. (2023). *Technofeudalism: What Killed Capitalism*. New York: Penguin Books.
Žižek, S. (1989). *The Sublime Object of Ideology*. London and New York: Verso.
Žižek, S. (1999). *The Ticklish Subject: The Absent Centre of Political Ontology*. London and New York: Verso.
Žižek, S. (2008). *In Defense of Lost Causes*. London and New York: Verso.
Žižek, S. (2025a). *Against Progress*. London and New York: Bloomsbury Academic.
Žižek, S. (2025b). *Zero Point*. London and New York: Bloomsbury Academic.
Zupančič, A. (2023). *Let Them Rot: Antigone's Parallax*. New York: Fordham University Press.

2 Situating proletariat discourse

The unconscious of capitalist discourse

An underlying argument of this chapter is that the proletariat discourse is positioned as a non-relationship or something that forms unconscious within Jacques Lacan's concept of capitalist discourse. Non-relationship refers to an element of thought that exists both within and outside discourse. It is inherent to the discourse but does not conform to it, illuminating a specific aspect of living beings. Capitalist discourse was introduced during the stage of late Lacan, a period of Lacan's psychoanalytic development that occurred after the event of May 1968 until his death in 1981. In this context, Karl Marx's concept of the proletariat is understood as a repressive substance that is ontologically inherent within Lacan's capitalist discourse. This location of the proletariat, which can be referred to as "a cause of desire" or something that is abandoned in the gaze framework (*objet a*) of the capitalist discourse, is not explicitly articulated by Lacan himself. While Lacan does not identify as a Marxist, the implications of the proletariat within Lacan's capitalist discourse give rise to a possibility to develop a proletariat discourse, which is constructed around four fundamental dimensions: psyche, existence, subject, and politics.

The chapter is organized into three main sections. The first section outlines Lacan's project on psychoanalytic discourse, which originated in 1969. Understanding psychoanalytic discourse is essential because Lacan's concept of capitalist discourse is framed within this broader context. From 1969 to 1971, during the period leading up to the development of capitalist discourse, Lacan, in his Seminar XVI, engages with Marx's discussion of the proletariat through the lens of surplus-value. He introduces his own concept of surplus-enjoyment (surplus-*jouissance*) to illuminate the capitalist subject and the consumerist individual within the realm of capitalist social objectivity (Lacan, 2024a, pp. 9–10). The second section focuses on capitalist discourse, which originated on May 12, 1972, in Milan. Lacan advises against interpreting capitalist discourse through a structuralist lens. Instead, he posits that the discourse functions as a signifier, where its representation of meaning alludes to another hidden, latent meaning

DOI: 10.4324/9781003657781-2

(Lacan 1978, pp. 32–55). This perspective hints at the position of the proletariat that Lacan recognizes, even though he does not explicitly articulate this dimension. The final section examines Lacan's critical suggestion regarding the need to transcend capitalist discourse. While an exit from capitalist discourse is deemed necessary, Lacan (1990, p. 16) warns against the potential misuse of his psychoanalysis to create a new form of sainthood without critically addressing the gap and ontological deficiency of the proletariat. Such an oversight could disrupt the teleological narrative of the revolutionary process.

A pre-production of the capitalist discourse: 1969–1971

A psychoanalytic discourse: the late Lacan's project

Lacan's understanding of the term "discourse" refers to an act of speech – the scheme in making the voice heard to exist in the universe of language (Lee, 2022, p. 125) – that aims to create a social bond. While this definition is widely accepted among Lacanian scholars and thinkers, it does not capture the full depth of Lacan's concept. Lacan emphasized that discourse, while forming a social bond, also contains elements that are "without speech", which suggests there is a "no point of closure" within discourse itself. To illustrate the tension between discourse and social bonds, Lacan uses the metaphor: "the pot has a hole in its homage" (Lacan, 2024a, p. 7).

In 1969, Lacan launched his psychoanalytic project entitled "A Psychoanalytic Discourse". During the first week of Seminar XVI, *From an Other to the other*, he illustrated this concept on the board by stating, "The essence of psychoanalytic theory is a discourse without speech" (Lacan, 2024a, pp. 3–6). This explanation echoes his earlier discussions on discourse from Seminar XIII, where he claimed, "There is no such thing as a universe of discourse". In both statements, discourse does not imply a total failure or a mere absence; instead, it signifies a characteristic of discourse that lacks "a point of closure" (Lacan, 2024a, p. 6). The idea of having no point of closure indicates that something remains unaddressed within the discourse itself, relating to the unconscious or the repressed substance that is inherent in every discourse (Moncayo et al., 2024, p. 191).

A general understanding of Lacan's discourse as a formation of social bonds is valid to some extent. However, it is important to also consider the mysterious nature of mute speech, including the repressed substance – essentially unspeakable – that is part of that social bond. Essentially, Lacan's true underlying discourse represents a social bond that does not fully achieve its intended purpose. In other words, the social bond reflects a fictionalization of reality. There exists an unconscious or repressed substance within the discourse that works against it, creating a gap where the discourse ultimately confronts its own wounds and reveals its disparities, as Lacan explains.

> The "truth's challenge to reality [*reel*]" is apparently relating to "the notion of the unconscious confronts us with a rule of thought that must be grounded on the basis of non-thought as something that could be its cause.
>
> (Lacan, 2024a, p. 5)

Lacan uses a gender term to metaphorize psychoanalytic discourse, stating that "psychoanalysis tells us that there is no union of man and woman" (Lacan, 2024a, p. 4). In this apparent union, there exists the unconscious, the "non-thought", and the essence of "something without speech", as he noted in a 1969 lecture, which serves to interrupt all discourse. He further asserts that "it is only to the extent that statements lie outside of meaning [*hors-de-sens*] – and not based on their meaning, as people think and as all of phenomenology assumes – that I am qua thought" (Lacan, 2024a, p. 5). In this assertion, Lacan suggests that the act of thinking is directed toward the unconscious, where meaning exists in a manner that is distinct from the foundational interpretations typically assumed by ordinary people and the field of phenomenology.

In brief, psychoanalytic discourse reveals that when Lacan examines each type of discourse, he does not view them simply as a formation of social bonds. Therefore, interpreting discourse solely as a reflection of the underlying truth and social connections is misleading, particularly in convergence with the influence of Hegelian dialectics on his psychoanalytic perspective.

The influence of Hegelian dialectics on Lacan's psychoanalytic discourse: a son killing two fathers?

Lacan once states that "*the death of structuralism, you are the son of Hegel.* I don't agree. I think in saying that Lacan *against* Hegel, you are much closer to the truth, though of course it is not at all a philosophical debate" (Lacan, 1981a, p. 215, italics original). But this does not mean that Hegelian dialectics does not play a significant role in Lacan's psychoanalytic discourse. André Green, a French psychoanalyst and colleague of Lacan, describes a relationship between Lacan and Hegel as that of a son who kills a father (Lacan, 1981a, p. 215). Lacan seems to embrace this characterization, suggesting that he, like a son, firstly imitates the behavior of his philosophical father, Hegel, only to eventually seek to "kill" him. Intriguingly, while Lacan acknowledges Hegel and considers him a master, he also positions Hegel as the target he aims to surpass. In this dynamic, Lacan presents himself as the hysterical Oedipal son who aspires to emulate the father before ultimately overcoming him. In addition to Green's observation, it can be extended nonetheless that Lacan is a son who may aspire to "kill two fathers", namely, Hegel and Marx.

Lacan, the son, begins his exploration without any hostility by following Hegel's principles of dialectics. It is untenable for an assertive discourse that claims to represent the semblance of truth to contain an inherent internal contradiction. There exists a gap between a discourse labeled as the semblance of truth and the actual occurrence of something that could dialectically dismantle it. In his project of psychoanalytic discourse, the late Lacan immediately identifies a dialectical image that is rooted in the semblance of truth laid within the signifier. He highlights this dialectical image's potential to disrupt the structural framework of discourse by referencing the ancient Jewish manuscripts known as the "Dead Sea Scrolls". He continues by stating, "The Dead Sea Scrolls, found in pots, remind us that it is not the signified that resides inside, but rather the signifier" (Lacan, 2024a, p. 8).

Despite the fact that the Dead Sea Scrolls are identified as a signifier, Lacan's statement does not intend to equate these Jewish manuscripts with a signifier. On the contrary, Lacan argues that the signifier fails in its overall function within a system of meaning because it is akin to a broken pot. Fortunately, a signifier can still convey some meaning to a certain extent. However, paradoxically, it also reveals its own limitations by leaving behind elements that remain non-signified in the realm of meaning. These non-signified elements are the significant images that interest Lacan. He points out that:

> Here we sense that the signification or image is truly on the outside, and that which is one the inside is precisely what lies in the grave where we find it – namely, precious materials and substances, perfumes, gold, frankincense, and myrrh.
>
> (Lacan, 2024a, p. 8)

The text above presents a nuanced argument that connects to a deeper understanding of the proletariat, comparable to the inner content of the Dead Sea Scrolls rather than its outer shell. It suggests that capitalist discourse serves as a pot, reminiscent of Lacan's idea of a pot that often has "a hole in its homage", as noted earlier. This analogy implies that the proletariat represents an unconscious aspect within the capitalist discourse that emerged in 1972. The emphasis of this 1972 capitalist discourse highlights the inherent lack and discontent experienced by capitalists. This perceived lack is necessary because it drives the capitalist subject to continually produce new products and commodities, striving to retain, reinvest, and regain profit. This is a circuit that leads to what Lacan calls a surplus-enjoyment. Since profit, money, and commodities are objects of unfulfilled desire, it is impossible for the capitalist subject to ever fully satisfy these cravings. Consequently, the capitalist subject seeks to cope, cover, and remedy this lack through surplus-enjoyment, which contributes to the ongoing expansion of capitalism as an existing reality.

Lacan's objective is not to outright oppose Marx's concept of surplus-value but rather to explore the psychoanalytic elements inherent in it. He approaches capitalist discourse from a psychoanalytic rather than an economic-theoretical standpoint. In this context, capitalist discourse serves as a means to reveal the unconscious thought processes of the capitalist subject. The essence of capitalist discourse can be compared to a clinical setting. Lacan positions himself as the psychoanalyst, while the capitalist subject assumes the role of the analysand, sharing their thoughts during the analysis. This dynamic resembles a session with Lacan, whose role is a doctor, investigating the capitalist subject as a thinking being. He seeks to delve into the subject's unconscious to bring it to light. Lacan poses a fundamental question: What occupies the mind of the capitalist subject, and what drives their relentless pursuit of profit accumulation? The psychoanalytic answer extends beyond the notion of surplus-value tied to exploitation and unpaid wages of labor in economic theory; it introduces the concept of surplus-enjoyment.

Surplus-enjoyment refers to the compulsive drive – one of the characteristics of the unconscious – that motivates capitalist subject to relentlessly pursue profit and introduce new commodities into the market. Given that capitalism is a dynamic system characterized by intense competition, it is essential for capitalist subject to experience a sense of lack, seek to remedy it, and fulfill this impossibility with a surplus-enjoyment. However, this situation gives rise to three key consequences, inevitably:

First, focusing on the unconscious dimension of capitalist subject leads to a psychoanalytic perspective of capitalism as a social reality that operates based on lack. In this view, the capitalist subject becomes a central figure in the pursuit of this social reality, in which a concrete form of it is a commodity and a market.

Second, this social reality enacted by capitalist subject is closely tied to the subjective experience of lack. It creates a sense of desire and need not only for capitalists but also for consumerist subject, fostering an addiction to a fetishism of consumption and a new mode of capitalist production (Tomšič, 2019; Vanheule, 2016; Alemán, 2024; Bruno, 2020; Swales, 2022). From a psychoanalytic standpoint, capitalism can be seen as the end of history, not only due to surplus-value but also because of surplus-enjoyment, which works in tandem with both objective and subjective lacks, including capitalist subject and consumerist subject.

However, the third point is crucial: capitalist discourse has to recognize the overlooked perspective that may initially seem external. It is a perspective that can be likened to what Lacan expresses as "precious materials and substances, perfumes, gold, frankincense, and myrrh", which lie beneath the surface of capitalist discourse, as mentioned earlier. This serves as a focal point for discussions about the proletariat discourse, which is ontologically positioned within the framework of capitalist discourse.

Following these three key consequences, the question arises: are the two fathers being killed or not? Hegelian dialectics reveal a paradox in every signifier, a concept that Lacan adopts from Hegel to highlight a gap in Marx's idea of surplus-value. Once this gap is identified, Lacan addresses it with his notion of capitalist discourse. This psychoanalytic dimension is something Marx overlooks due to his fixation on language within economic theory. Lacan aims to surpass Hegel's ideas because Hegel does not apply the principles of dialectics in a psychoanalytic manner, particularly regarding his psychoanalytic invention of capitalist discourse. At this juncture, Lacan, representing an Oedipal hysterical son, begins to challenge and, in a sense, "kill" the father figure of Hegel. The next potential target is Marx, as a second father figure. Whether Lacan views Marx as a father figure remains uncertain, but it is plausible that he attempts to challenge or override Marx's concept of surplus-value with his psychoanalytic invention of surplus-enjoyment, a concept that is well recognized among Lacanian-Marxist scholars today. Ultimately, despite the symbolic "killing" of these two fathers, Lacan's psychoanalytic discourse continues to focus on the function of the *objet a*.

Introducing **objet a***: from the object cause of desire to the being of non-relationship in every discourse*

The concept of *objet a* is indispensable for discussing capitalist discourse. It highlights the presence of both the capitalist subject and the consumerist subject while revealing the absent unconscious that remains invisible at the center of capitalist discourse, specifically the proletariat. Moreover, understanding how *objet a* is developed historically by Lacan is crucial as it reveals how this term functions significantly within Lacanian psychoanalysis.

To begin with, the early Lacan describes *objet a* in Seminar VII. The notion refers to the "object cause of desire", which is often seen as the site that Lacan designates literally as "impassable", or "as the side of the Thing" (Lacan, 2008a, p. 263). According to the early stage of Lacan's thought, this object cause of desire could be elevated to the special status of the Thing. This status exists outside a moral imperative of reality principle. While society may perceive it as another site of impossible desire, the subject considers it to be achievable (Lacan, 2008b, pp. 135–139). This classical interpretation has gained popularity within the Lacanian community and is rooted in early Lacan's work.

During the mid-phase of Lacan's work, particularly in Seminar XI, Lacan further develops the concept of *objet a* by examining the complex relationship within the field of vision. Here, *objet a* emerges as a desirable object that is inherently present within the framework yet appears to be absent from one's direct sight: the existence of the being of non-relationship in every discourse. This notion can be viewed from two perspectives. First, *objet a* suggests an absence or something that is missing within the field of vision. The gaze perceives the subject from a place that the subject himself is not aware of. This aspect of *objet a* aligns with Lacan's description: "it was looking at me at the level of the point of light, the point at which everything that looks at me is situated" (Lacan, 1981b, p. 95). Thus, *objet a* is already located within the field of vision, but the subject dismisses it, even while being positioned within the same framework. Second, Lacan explores a different scenario. In the context of the relationship between the subject as a spectator and the picture, the subject's gaze can be understood as *objet a* because "the picture, certainly, is in my eye. But I am not in the picture" (Lacan, 1981b, p. 96). The picture fails to acknowledge the subject's gaze internal to the picture, as if it exists outside the framework. This leads Lacan to emphasize that "you never look at me from the place I see you" (Lacan, 1981b, p. 91). Ironically, "the picture is certainly in my eye, but I am not in the picture" (Lacan, 1981b, p. 96). The gaze, as the depicted object becomes unrepresented, embodies a lost yet desirable object that fuels desire, despite being ultimately excluded from the framework of perception, perspective, and gaze.

Lacan's discussion of the gaze and *objet a* becomes a foundational concept for approaching the painting *Las Meninas* (1656), as presented in his Seminar XIII (Lacan, 1966a). Based on the painting, one can explore how the subjects, particularly the King and the Queen, are depicted within the painting. These royal figures are portrayed as central subjects by the artist Diego Velázquez; however, their placement outside the direct line of public gaze creates a sense of being unframed. While the focus of public attention is primarily on Margarita Teresa, the five-year-old infanta who is considered the central figure, this emphasis highlights the disconnect experienced by "the pictured" figures who are ignored by the public gaze. The King and the Queen exemplify this grotesque element of the being of non-relationship – present yet removed from a perspectival gaze – which disrupts the entire visual frame and leads to a division in the discourse surrounding the painting. This sense of non-relationship can disturb public discourse, particularly public opinion and consciousness, prompting the spectator to seek the object cause of desire outside the gaze framework: the *objet a*.

In Seminar XIV (Lacan, 1966b), Lacan's overall objective is a critique of the notion of fantasy, arguing that the Other, which is the field of language and its objective apparatus, informs individuals about what to desire. As a result, people often accept these desires as their own without critical reflection. This unexamined or imprudent acceptance of desire leads to a fantasy that shapes the subject's cause of desire in a perverse manner. Lacan likens the function of fantasy to a vast machine of desire that tells individuals what to want. He uses the metaphor of a lozenge: individuals consume it, enjoying its sweet taste as the object that generates their excitement without seeking alternatives to this intoxicating desire. Ultimately, individuals remain in a state of perversion unless they cease to cooperate with the Other – a delusional social bond maintained through fantasy that upholds a misleading reality.

The most significant aspect of Lacan's concept of *objet a,* developed from his middle to late work, is that it represents the unconscious, the being of non-relationship, which is inherently present in every discourse, even in fantasies, which are fundamentally a perverse form of desire. In Lacan's critique of fantasy, it is suggested that fantasies operate in tandem with "the desire of the Other". It is crucial to recognize that there is always a remainder that creates a gap within the realm of fantasy. The formula for understanding fantasy is, unsurprisingly, represented as $ <> a. To clarify this: first, fantasy equates to the concept of the Other, but in terms of desire, this can be misleading. Second, the individual, regardless of being a man or woman, positioned before the Other is represented as the barred subject ($). This is because they become perverse by failing to accurately inquire into what they truly desire. Lastly, at the end of this formula, there is the *a*, which stands for *objet a*. Lacan refers to this *objet a* to emphasize that there is something that could potentially disrupt the entire realm of fantasy. He aims to outline something that is mystically desirable yet is not identical to the realm of fantasy. This absolute remainder acts as the *objet a*, the being of non-relationship that exists in every discourse, that the subject has to connect to it. It is simultaneously the element absent from the gaze framework. However, seeking, identifying, and connecting with it is not impossible. This is crucial for understanding Lacan's introduction of capitalist discourse in 1972 and for engaging critically with Marx, particularly regarding the capitalist subject, surplus-value, surplus-enjoyment, and, above all, the proletariat. At this point, it is essential to examine how *objet a* plays a critical role in two dimensions – *the two theses of objet a* – particularly in relation to capitalism, in the late Lacan.

The first thesis on objet a*: the capitalist subject, surplus-enjoyment, and masochistic subject*

During the feudal era, capitalists were subjects whose power was subordinate to that of the monarchy and aristocrats. However, as the influence of monarchy faded, capitalists began to emerge as active subjects, dominating the era of industrialization and digitalization. From an economic theory perspective, capitalists are individuals who own the means of production and utilize it for business growth and profit accumulation. However, from a psychoanalytic perspective, a capitalist subject embodies what Sigmund Freud refers to as the vividity and enthusiasm of something that is capable of becoming actively conscious from the negative point of repression (Freud, 2010, p. 3).

Nonetheless, defining capitalist subject solely as a Freudian return of the repressed individual overlooks a Lacanian perspective pertaining to capitalist subject's relationship with the concepts of surplus-enjoyment and masochism. Therefore, the first thesis on *objet a* focuses on the capitalist subject's preoccupation with surplus-enjoyment, which is a condition for the capitalist subject to turn also into masochism. It is relevant to begin this section with a passage quoted directly from Lacan:

> I will call on Marx, who it was hard for me – bothered as I was about it for a long time – not to bring sooner in a field where he certainly has his place. As Marx does [regarding surplus value], I will indicate the place where we must situate the essential function of *objet a*.
>
> (Lacan, 2024a, p. 8)

In retrospect, Marx's concept of surplus-value (*Mehrwert*) highlights that the benefits gained by the proletariat are less than the value of the labor they provide. Lacan continues to analyze Marx's notion of surplus-value, stating,

> what is new in his approach is how he situates labor. It is not that labor is a new concept, but rather that it is purchased and that there is a market for labor. This allows Marx to illustrate what is innovative in his discourse: surplus-value.
>
> (Lacan, 2024a, p. 8)

Yet, in the statement above, it is seen that Lacan introduces *objet a*, which represents the inherent non-relationship found in every discourse. He seems to caution that there is a disruptive element at the core of this discourse that could challenge Marx's understanding of surplus-value. In this context, what does *objet a* signify? In response, Lacan identifies it as the "capitalist subject" (Lacan, 2024a, p. 8) in relation to the capitalist organization of production, distribution, and commodification. In other words, to grasp the role of *objet a* in this discussion, Lacan describes it as the capitalist subject. He points out to Marxist audiences that "you are not very familiar with this term", suggesting that the concept of the capitalist subject may seem strange or atypical to them (Lacan, 2024a, p. 8). Thus, in the context of a discussion, the first thesis on *objet a* is embodied in the capitalist subject.

As a psychoanalyst interested in exploring the thoughts of the capitalist subject, Lacan employs the German term *Mehrlust*, which translates to over-enjoyment. He equates this concept with surplus-enjoyment, also known as surplus-*jouissance* or *plus-de-jouir*. Lacan's aim is to explore the desires of the capitalist subject. Importantly, the function of the *objet a* not only pertains to the capitalist subject but also aids in understanding surplus-enjoyment. This introduces a psychoanalytic dimension that Marx's concept of surplus-value does not address. It is not entirely convincing to equate Marx's *Mehrwert* directly with Lacan's *Mehrlust*. Lacan himself cautions against this assumption, stating in his own words, "I thus attached, superimposed, and plastered the notion of surplus *jouissance* [*plus-de-jouir*] onto the flipside of surplus value" (Lacan, 2024c, p. 19). He certainly elaborates on the relationship between these two concepts as homologous, while also recognizing the complexities and limitations that this homology presents (Lacan, 2024c, p. 19). A more precise interpretation of Lacan's intention is that his concept of *Mehrlust* serves as the *objet a* in relation to Marx's *Mehrwert*.

The theoretical comparison between Lacan and Marx often overlooks the history of interpreting Marx's work within the French context. This re-framing of Marx within the French context strengthens and deepens Lacan's critical understanding of Marx. Elisabeth Roudinesco notes that during the 1964–1965 academic year, there was a study group that focused on Marx's *Capital* that aimed to provide Marx with a "symptomatic reading or interpretation" (Roudinesco, 2005, p. 306). The intention is not to interpret Marx's work in a literal, biblical sense but rather to identify a symptom within Marx's text. Roudinesco (2005) notes that "the aim was to bring out what was untranslatable and unthought in Marx's work and to separate the texts of his youth, still showing traces of Hegel and the category of the subject" (p. 306). It is this French context that specifically inspires Lacan's own revisions not only of Freud but also of Marx.

Lacan and Marx share both points of agreement and disagreement, rather than a sense of harmony. While both thinkers critique capitalism, Lacan revises Marx's concept of surplus-value by shifting it to a different perspective. Instead of viewing it as an absolute fatality, he highlights its limitations and gaps. By introducing the absent element into Marx's discourse, Lacan reveals an important aspect: the capitalist subject's connection to surplus-enjoyment. This relationship ultimately leads to the impossibility of fulfilling desire (Bianchi, 2010, pp. 123–137). This issue corresponds with Seminar XVI, where Lacan suggests that surplus-enjoyment pertains to capitalist and consumerist subjects. It particularly addresses their economic activities in a consumer society characterized by commodification, distribution, excessive consumption, and an unending drive for accumulation.

In addition to experiencing surplus-enjoyment, the capitalist subject can also be understood as a masochistic subject. This connection arises because the capitalist subject is, in reality, successful in attaining enjoyment. However, this subject pretends that their enjoyment is somehow unfulfilled and significantly diminished. By doing so, they create a fantasy of lack, which serves as a useful psychical mechanism that drives them to seek even greater, excessive pleasure. In the context of masochism, this sense of lack becomes a constant psychological tool for creating fantasy. It is this masochistic fantasy that encourages individuals to chastise themselves for feeling inadequate, motivating them to pursue more intense pleasures beyond their current experiences in order to cope with their perceived lack. Samo Tomšic (2015, p. 229) suggests that the masochism experienced by the capitalist subject reflects a tendency to perceive lack as a self-inflicted condition. The masochistic subject deliberatively links pleasure with feelings of insufficiency, leading them to continually seek more pleasure while ultimately diminishing it to a zero level. It is this condition, characterized by a self-perception of almost total lack of enjoyment, that allows the masochistic capitalist subject to obsess over excessive, surplus-enjoyment.

Furthermore, Andreja Zevnik suggests that in Lacan's article "Kant with Sade", masochism is essential for understanding the relationship between capitalism and the psychoanalytic concept of castration (Zevnik, 2022, p. 42). In this article, Lacan implies that instead of simply forfeiting, he seeks to redefine castration by linking it to the fantasy of the masochistic subject. Lacan refers to this as "a Sadean fantasy" (Lacan, 2006a, pp. 653–665). In this context, castration is no longer viewed as a conventional external factor that normatively imposes an actual prohibition on the subject's desires. Instead, it takes on a new significance; castration becomes useful for the fantasy surrounding the subject's sense of lack and an active pursuit of surplus-enjoyment. Here, the fantasy of castration is seen as a means for the subject's "will to *jouissance*" (Lacan, 2006a, p. 654). Castration indicates that the subject acts as a self-cause, agreeing to be motivated by a virtual castration that leads to a fantasy of unfulfilled desires beyond certain limits. From the perspective of the masochistic subject, this fantasy indicates consent to the tormentor's intentions. Therefore, the belief in the existence of castration serves as a condition for enhancing enjoyment for the masochist (Lacan, 2006a, p. 665). To clarify further, this is not solely a forfeiture of castration; rather, it reveals a new dimension of castration that is not tied to the Oedipus complex. Instead, it relates to the subject of masochism actively imposing a virtual castration of desire upon themselves.

The concept of masochism is closely linked to the structure and dynamics of capitalism. This connection is represented by the masochistic subject, who deliberately rejects enjoyment to maintain a form of self-torment. This rejection creates a distorted sense of lack, actively driving the masochistic subject – such as the capitalist subject – to maintain and seek greater, excessive, or surplus-enjoyment. In other words, while the capitalist subject may achieve enjoyment, it appears as if they deliberately diminish their level of enjoyment to connect with their sense of lack. This experience of enjoying lack becomes a condition for seeking more excessive enjoyment. Thus, reducing the capitalist subject to merely being a return of the repressed is insufficient. When using a masochistic logic to analyze capitalism, it is important to recognize that capitalist subject often engages in the fantasy of lack. Lacan suggests that for the capitalist subject, "this function appears owing to the very existence of discourse. It demonstrates that the renunciation of *jouissance* is an effect of discourse itself" (Lacan, 2024a, p. 9). When considering a capitalist subject as a masochistic subject, their surplus-enjoyment "arises from the renunciation of *jouissance* owing to the effect of discourse" (Lacan, 2024a, p. 10). This observation highlights a crucial point: Lacan's concept of surplus-enjoyment is essential for understanding the desire of the capitalist subject, and the psychoanalytic aspects of how capitalism operates, a dimension of thought that does not entirely oppose but is often neglected in the context of surplus-value in Marx's theory.

The second thesis on* objet a*: the speculative truth of the proletariat is neither a surplus-value nor surplus-enjoyment

In the second thesis regarding *objet a*, Lacan's focus appears to direct his attention to the proletariat. Instead of placing and integrating the proletariat into the entropic theoretical frameworks associated with Marx's surplus-value, he shifts the discussion away from his own concept of surplus-enjoyment. To begin with, it is important to reflect Lacan's statement:

> Regarding recourse to *jouissance* – in which, due to the sign, something else occupies its place, namely, the trait that marks it – nothing is identifiable. Nothing can arise here without an object being lost.
>
> (Lacan, 2024a, p. 12)

From the passage, Lacan discusses the existence of the internal contradiction inherent in discourse and the ontology of discourse associated with the ineluctable cleavage. He argues that every discourse contains a signifier that possesses an opaque element, which complicates interpretation over the passage. Recourse to surplus-enjoyment or *jouissance*, there is an opacity. This opacity leads to a recognition of an "object being lost", referred to at the same time as a "non-identifiable" object. Rather than representing an ideal, this lost object embodies a material reality of "something else" that replaces the state of surplus-enjoyment enacted by the capitalist subject. This missing object, which is absent from our gaze, is known as the *objet a*. As there is something characterized as the non-identifiable and the object being lost at the state of surplus-enjoyment, it is suggested that this opaque object may symbolize the position of the proletariat, as it is the capitalist, not the proletariat, who occupies the position of surplus-enjoyment.

The interpretation of the lost object, which relates to the implications of the proletariat, raises some interesting considerations. Lacan elaborates on this in the following two sentences. In the first sentence, he states,

> Here the subject is stifled and effaced at the very moment he appears. How can some aspect of this subject, which disappears as soon as he emerges, created by a signifier only to immediately fade in another, be constituted and ultimately achieve a sense of self-consciousness or self-awareness? In other words, how can it become something that is satisfied with being identical to itself? This is what we must now consider.
>
> (Lacan, 2024a, p. 12)

In the second sentence, Lacan considers and clarifies the position of the stifled and effaced subject by illuminating that "it is in the gap between exchange value and use value that what is known as surplus-value arises and fades away" (Lacan, 2024a, p. 12). This suggests that proletariat could be symbolized as surplus-value while simultaneously being effaced from that symbolization because the proletariat is not "satisfied with being identical" to such symbolization.

In other words, the proletariat is seen primarily as something that should be identical to itself, representing what used to occupy the place of surplus-value. However, the proletariat cannot remain stagnant in this position as an exploited labor force. If it does, it risks becoming a subject that disappears, fades away, and fails to achieve self-consciousness or self-awareness. The subject cannot allow itself to experience such a transcendental loss; as a result, proletariat becomes "no longer identical to itself, the subject no longer enjoys" (Lacan, 2024a, pp. 12–13). This implies that something essential is lost and no longer enjoys surplus-enjoyment. It is the proletariat that represents a subject that is emptied of surplus-enjoyment and "no longer enjoys", as this position of surplus-enjoyment is reserved for the capitalist subject.

This is where the second thesis on *objet a* is invoked to fulfill its purpose. Lacan emphasizes the point that "in the definition of the subject as caused by the relationship between signifiers, we have theoretically posited – a priori and without any – something that prohibits us from ever grasping him" (Lacan, 2024a, p. 13). In this statement, it can be argued that the subject refers to the proletariat. Lacan's phrase "something that prohibits us from ever grasping him" suggests a specific position of the "I" within the system. This "I" indicates a departure from the capitalist subject, which naturally leads us to the second thesis of *objet a*. The *objet a* represents "something else" that "prohibits us from ever grasping him", an element that eludes both surplus-value and surplus-enjoyment.

To clarify, the question being explored is: what is the "something else" that "prohibits us from ever grasping him"? The answer lies in the proletariat. Lacan uncovers this answer, indicating by himself, literally, that "when this 'I' is in the place of the *worker*, which is ever more generally the case, the position implies demanding something related to worker's frustration" (Lacan, 2024c, p. 26, italics original). Furthermore, Lacan elaborates on the frustration of the worker as leading to "the small reconstructions that are characterized as 'revolutions'" (Lacan, 2024c, p. 27). Thus, in his words:

> The worker inscribes himself qua "I". I am saying "I". Note that I did not say "subject", whereas I mentioned the capitalist subject.
>
> (Lacan, 2024c, p. 26)

In this statement, the "I" refers to the worker, or the proletariat, and the "subject" also represents the "I", which is the proletariat. None of these references mentions the capitalist subject. This implies that Lacan's concept of the proletariat is neither a surplus-enjoyment experienced by the capitalist subject in its interaction with its own fantasy of lack in the market economy nor is it a surplus-value that pertains to the exploited labor. Furthermore, another clue that one gathers from closely reading Lacan's instruction is revealed in the following sentence:

> The worker Is undoubtedly the sacred site of the conceptual element that constitutes the truth of the system, and that emerges when knowledge – which holds together all the more perfectly because it is identical to its own precept in being – rips apart somewhere. . . . Let us see what this structural fabric feels like, and cut it with our scissors.
>
> (Lacan, 2024c, p. 27)

In the statement above, the proletariat is seen as "sacred site" that reveals the truth of the system by the act of tearing apart the structural fabric devised by a system of capitalism. Within this structural fabric, whether it involves surplus-value or surplus-enjoyment, if the proletariat remains voiceless, there will be no truth about their condition. Lacan's notion of "our scissors" suggests that the proletariat can cut off and resist the capitalist system, but this understanding must be approached with caution. Lacan discusses the proletariat in the same sense as Marx's proletariat in the following:

> It just so happens that excess exploitation displeases people. I say "displeases people" because there is nothing further to be said about it. The principle of revolutionary revolt is none other than the fact that there is a point at which things displease people.
>
> (Lacan, 2024b, p. 307)

While Lacan appears to advocate for the proletariat as a revolutionary agency, one should refrain from categorizing him strictly as a Marxist, as he seems to harbor skepticism toward Marx's conception of the proletariat as well.

Lacan is interested in examining the speculative truth of the proletariat itself. He explores the relationship between the proletariat and its self-inquiry regarding this truth. In this context, the proletariat, understood as a speculative truth, has to avoid becoming entangled in surplus-enjoyment and surplus-value. According to Lacan, the proletariat has the audacity to identify itself with "the master's philosophy". However, its lack of this speculative truth about itself arises from how the proletariat perceives itself, particularly in relation to surplus-enjoyment and surplus-value. To revitalize the concept of the proletariat as a speculative truth, one could draw on Lacan's insights about the subject:

> Prior to that, the proletariat – as the master's philosophy, which was the first, had the gall to call it – had the right to do what you know: abstain. As you hear in misleading places designed for this precise purpose, if I dare say so,

> psychoanalysis simply ignores class struggle. This is perhaps not entirely clear, for psychoanalysis could even give back its true meaning.
>
> (Lacan, 2024d, p. 344)

The sentence above highlights that the proletariat, which occupies the realm of the master's philosophy, boldly identifies with that position and, paradoxically, has the right to refrain from taking action, unless they become firstly independent of the concepts – surplus-enjoyment and surplus-value – that seek to determine it. In some misleading contexts, it can be argued that psychoanalysis overlooks class struggle. However, this assertion may not be entirely accurate, as psychoanalysis could potentially restore the true meaning of class struggle. Lacan clearly emphasizes to the proletariat that "psychoanalysis could give it back its true meaning". However, it is important not to hastily conclude that Lacanian psychoanalysis is entirely synonymous with the Marxist concept of class struggle, nor should one simplistically label Lacan as a Marxist.

Why is it inappropriate to categorize and label Lacan primarily as Marxist? Although Lacan explicitly states that psychoanalysis could reconnect with and ultimately preserve a genuine understanding of the class struggle for the proletariat, this political aspect of class struggle does not fully capture the broader speculative truth concerning the proletariat. Class struggle is just one element of the broader speculative truth about the proletariat. This raises significant concerns, as it does not fully capture the complexities of the proletariat in itself as viewed through Lacan's psychoanalysis. In other words, a deeper and more critical analysis of the proletariat from a Lacanian perspective may be necessary for Lacan's ideas to build upon Marx's original insights regarding the proletariat.

This, in consequence, promulgates the proletariat in divergence of a scientific knowledge that governs them, or, in a typical Lacanian manner, it represents the proletariat negating its identity as embodied in the figure of the "science's man" (Lacan, 2006c, p. 730). Lacan interprets Vladimir Lenin's metaphysical conception of proletariat consciousness, along with his ideal image of a dictatorship aimed at establishing a proletariat state, as a splitting (*Spaltung*) from the speculative truth of the proletariat. According to Lacan, Lenin's discourse on Marx's theory, along with the Leninist imaginary of the proletariat, represents the master philosophy regarding the proletariat, to which this image of proletariat as a man of science leads to the silencing of the proletariat's own voice (Lacan, 2006c, p. 738). Lacan critiques Lenin's concept of class consciousness by implying the proletariat as a psychoanalytical embodiment of the speculative truth that transcends the limitations imposed by scientific knowledge. This criticism highlights a fundamental distinction between the knowledge about the proletariat, which represents a certain truth from Lenin's perspective, and the speculative truth of the proletariat itself, which Lacan considers a possible form of abstract purity. In essence, Lacan's viewpoint asserts that the essence of the proletariat cannot be reduced to mere scientific representation. This does not mean that psychoanalysis negates science. Instead, it can be considered a science only to the extent that it challenges the unified narrative imposed by scientific discourse. While science often presents a singular body of knowledge such as Lenin's discourse on the proletariat, psychoanalysis seeks to address elements that lie beyond what has already been written. This elusive aspect, which cannot be dismissed, represents an aspect of truth and science that Lacanian psychoanalysis endorses (Lacan, 1973).

Lacan's critique of Lenin's portrayal of the proletariat prompts an examination of the distinction between proletariat as the "I", or "the subject does" (Lacan, 2006c, p. 730), and the scientific understanding of proletariat exemplified in Lenin's overdetermined discourse. This ontological gap in a proletariat subject can also be articulated through the fundamental difference between proletariat portrayed in the idea of "where it was, there must I come to be as a subject" ("*Wo Es war, soll Ich werden*") (Lacan, 2006d, p. 347) and the notion that castrates and annihilates the proletariat as "I" as a subject, which is represented by Lenin's royal science of the proletariat, or, the proletariat allocated in a discourse of the science of man.

In his essay "Science and Truth" (1966), Lacan's denial of the science of man is clear; he states, "there is no such thing as a science of man because science's man does not exist; only its subject does" (Lacan, 2006c, p. 730). Thus, the phrase "the subject does" refers to the proletariat as "I", which speaks as such, contrasting with the proletariat being orchestrated as a subject of science. The scientific knowledge representation of the proletariat is characterized as "the lack of truth about truth", which fails to display "the truth about truth". In other words, the speculative truth of the proletariat reveals that the dominant truth about them, shaped by scientific knowledge, leads to a fundamental repression (*Urverdrängung*). This repression serves as a mechanism of knowledge that obscures – by creating an unconscious blind spot – the essence of the proletariat as a psychoanalytic being that encompasses the psyche, existence, subjectivity, and politics: the four fundamental dimensions of the proletariat discourse as mentioned in the introductory chapter. At this unconscious blind spot, which stands in opposition to the science of man, a Lacanian psychoanalytic view of the proletariat suggests that it possesses its own "some-Thing else" (*Autre Chose*).

For Lacan, aligning with Spinoza, this expression of "some-Thing else" resembles the Spinozian concept of self-cause. Therefore, individuals, or the proletariat in this case, must seek to discover and ultimately embody their potential as "a God in Man". Although this notion may seem blasphemous, a Lacanian-Marxist perspective interprets God as embodied within each person, positioning the proletariat as a divine entity in its own right. Importantly, this conception of God does not succumb to the pantheistic idea of God (Lacan, 2006c, p. 735).

What is the speculative truth of the proletariat? How does the proletariat determine a self-cause within itself? According to Lacan, prior to 1972, the proletariat is neither surplus-value nor surplus-enjoyment, as neither conveys the embodiment of the self-cause of the proletariat. Additionally, the essence of the proletariat transcends Lenin's framework. Psychoanalytically, the proletariat expresses truth – as the "I", as the "subject that acts", as "*Wo Es war, soll Ich werden*", and as "some-Thing else" – only to the extent that this speculative truth about proletariat broadens the formation of class consciousness that is regulated by Leninist ideology, which seeks to establish a dictatorial government of the proletariat. Lacan continues that "it might not be bad to remind you that Marxist theory, inasmuch as it concerns a truth, in fact states that the truth of capitalism is the proletariat. That's true: it is a truth" (Lacan, 2024e, p. 148). Ultimately, Lacan's critique differentiates Lenin's discourse on the proletariat in two categories: the proletariat that embodies the class consciousness of a political party, where genuine truth is seldom spoken, and the proletariat in itself, who acts as a savant, and who begins to realize the truth for himself. This distinction means that the proletariat in itself should not be reduced to the party that rarely articulates the truth about it:

> What is meant by proletariat? It means that work is reduced to a pure and simple commodity, which means that the worker himself is reduced to the same status [i.e., he is just another commodity]. But as soon as the worker learns that about himself, thanks to the theory, we can say that, owing to this step, he finds pathways to a status – call it as you will – qua savant. He is no longer part of the proletariat *an sich* [in itself], as it were; he is no longer a pure and simple truth; he is *für sich* [for himself], he is what is known as "class consciousness." And he may even simultaneously become the class consciousness of a party in which no one ever speaks the truth again.
>
> (Lacan, 2024e, p. 148)

The birth of the capitalist discourse: May 12, 1972

Lacan's capitalist discourse was introduced at the University of Milan on May 12, 1972 (Lacan, 1978, pp. 32–55). To understand Lacan's capitalist discourse, it is essential to refer to his own words, as they are considered a legitimate primary source. Notably, his speech at the University of Milan serves as a key resource for grasping the concept of capitalist discourse. This work was eventually published in 1978 as a bilingual volume titled "Discours de Jacques Lacan à l'Université de Milan le 12 mai 1972, paru dans l'ouvrage bilingue" by *La Salamandra*.

This section will build on the mentioned work, arguing that capitalist discourse not only addresses the capitalist subject and the surplus-enjoyment associated with it but also implies the presence of the proletariat. To gain a comprehensive understanding of Lacan's concept of capitalist discourse, it is beneficial to analyze his Milan speech into two sections. In the first section, Lacan explains his project called psychoanalytic discourse and its relation to the shifts in meaning or sliding within the signifier. In the second section, he presents a diagram of capitalist discourse, describing it as an inversion of his master discourse. He emphasizes that capitalist discourse should not be interpreted solely through a structuralist lens. This perspective allows the proletariat, seen as the unconscious within this discourse, to emerge and be acknowledged.

First section: proletariat as a "slippage within the signifier"

At the beginning of the lecture, Lacan introduces his project by stating, "I announced that I would speak about Psychoanalytic Discourse – it is not a term that I have put forward for a long time – but still for three years" (Lacan, 1978, p. 33: my translation). This is not surprising for those who closely follow Lacan's work. As mentioned in the previous section of this chapter, Lacan initiated the project known as psychoanalytic discourse in 1969 during Seminar XVI, prior to 1972. It is important to emphasize that capitalist discourse is incorporated into his project of psychoanalytic discourse (Lacan, 1978, p. 49: my translation).

Lacan explains that he identifies four main types of psychoanalytic discourse: master discourse, university discourse, hysteric discourse, and analyst discourse. He also includes capitalist discourse as a fifth discourse (see Figure 2.1). In the diagram, the top left represents the position of the "agency", indicating those who actively perform an action. The bottom left represents the "truth" of the discourse. The top right designates the "other", or anyone who is related to or subordinated by the agency, while the bottom right addresses the "production" or

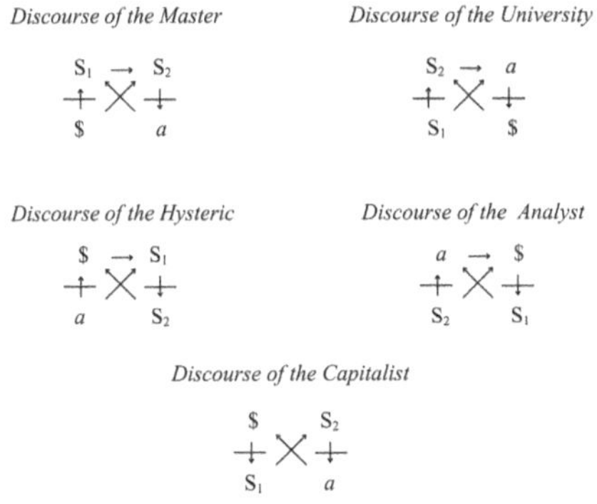

Figure 2.1 The five discourses.

Source: Figure adapted from Daniela, D., and Carlos Gomez Camarena. (2022). 'Annex II. What is *matheme*? Four Discourses and Mathematics in Lacan', in *The Marx Through Lacan Vocabulary: A Compass for Libidinal and Political Economies*. Edited by Christina Soto Van Der Plas et al. London and New York: Routledge. p. 289.

the effects produced by the agency on others. Lacan cautions anyone seeking to understand his five discourses about the complexity and elusiveness of signifiers. For instance, master discourse is not limited to a simple master-slave relationship; it can also suggest a lack of knowledge on the part of the master regarding the slave. The master can take on the role of the analyst, and conversely, can slide into a hysterical position. Another example is capitalist can represent the master, with corporate CEOs exemplifying this role. Capitalists often dominate university discourse by influencing the design of university curricula. They may also adopt a hysterical position by creating new technologies that disrupt existing capitalist organizations and production processes. Furthermore, capitalists can act as analysts by analyzing customer desires and needs. Ultimately, these examples illustrate the fluidity of signifiers and how one can shift into another.

Each signifier inevitably encounters what Lacan refers to as "the slippage within the signifier" (Lacan, 1978, p. 36: my translation). In Lacan's view, "what I will call is the game of signifiers. The game of signifiers slips into meaning. But the imperative of what I am saying is that it never slips except in the form of a skid" (Lacan, 1978, p. 35: my translation). This sliding occurs within the mechanism of the signifier itself. Specifically, this suggests that there is always something slipping away from the signifier's mechanism. However, this elusive element is not without value; instead, it signifies a crucial aspect of being. Thus, being is something concealed within the signifier; it conceals itself in the language used to represent things. Lacan emphasizes that "the word being has no meaning outside of language" (Lacan, 1978, p. 36: my translation).

Ultimately, when Lacan discusses the signifier of capitalist discourse, he aims to highlight not just the capitalist subject but also to acknowledge a slippage in the signifier – specifically, the being that exists within language itself, which implies the location of the proletariat. According to Lacan, "it is language that messed everything up" (Lacan, 1978, p. 39: my translation). This suggests that the language of capitalist discourse can confuse anyone who believes that the focus of a discourse is solely on the capitalist subject. However, this perspective is misleading. Such thinking risks overlooking the unconscious aspects of capitalist discourse, where the proletariat represents the being of that unconscious.

Second section: capitalist discourse, proletariat, and a departure from a structuralist interpretation

In the latter part of the lecture, Lacan introduces the concept of capitalist discourse, referring to it as "something crazy clever" (Lacan, 1978, p. 48: my translation). He explains that capitalist discourse represents a slight inversion of master discourse. Specifically, on the left side of the diagram, both the upper and lower columns of capitalist discourse show "a very small inversion simply between the S_1 and the \$, which is the subject" (Lacan, 1978, p. 48: my translation) compared to master discourse. This subtle shift is what leads Lacan to describe capitalist discourse as exceptionally "crazy clever" discourse.

Based on Lacan's original insight, his capitalist discourse does not seek to align harmoniously with Marx's theories. Lacan explicitly states that in critiquing capitalism, "Marx teaches them [Marxists] that what is involved is only surplus-value" (Lacan, 1978, p. 49: my translation). He immediately adds that there is a psychoanalytical structure related to a capitalist subject that Marx is likely to overlook, as indicated in his remark, "it's added enjoyment . . . eh?" (Lacan, 1978, p. 49: my translation), which refers to surplus-enjoyment.

Lacan explains that "what I call surplus-enjoyment, because it is the term that is applied to this level, which we know well, which is called desire" (Lacan, 1978, p. 51: my translation). Desire is obscure as it points to a cause of desire, which is called by Lacan the *objet a*. With the introduction of the *objet a* into the discussion, the capitalist subject, who often embodies masochistic characteristics, intends to experience a constant sense of lack and never achieves true satisfaction, as previously mentioned in the earlier section.

The effect of the *objet a* invigorates the capitalist subject to have an incessant drive to tie their lives to "a very beautiful object" (Lacan, 1978, p. 52: my translation), such as profit, power, and prosperity. This leads them to become "accustomed to sucking" (Lacan, 1978, p. 52: my translation). As a result, it seems that the capitalist subject "sucks like that all their lives" (Lacan, 1978, p. 52: my translation) by negating satisfaction. In this sense, the capitalist subject can be seen as a masochistic being that "it consumes itself so well that it consumes itself" (Lacan, 1978, p. 48: my translation), in a remarkable and endless manner in this maze of capitalism. Ultimately, Lacan's perspective on capitalist discourse presents a critical stance toward capitalism without resorting to Marx's surplus-value. He questions, "What is discourse?" and asserts that it acts as a social bond, but personally, he does not believe in it (Lacan, 1978, p. 51: my translation). This suggests that while Lacan may agree with Marx's notion of surplus-value to some extent, he ultimately disagrees with it by revealing a psychoanalytic dimension known as surplus-enjoyment. This idea will become clearer in the framework of capitalist discourse, but to fully understand capitalist discourse, it is suggested to first examine the master discourse.

Master discourse illustrates a dialectic between the master and the slave. In a diagram (see Figure 2.1), it begins with the master or agency (S_1) positioned at the top left, whose action is to dominate the slave located at the top right (S_2). At the bottom left, there exists the truth in the form of a divided subject ($) representing the slave. Additionally, the production or product of the discourse reveals a cause of desire (a), which acts as a surplus regarding the knowledge of the slave itself, in addition to $. In contrast, capitalist discourse blurs the lines between master and slave, suggesting that they are, in fact, the same individuals. In this view, the distinction between agency and slave is erased. This corresponds with Lacan's observation that capitalist discourse is a "crazy clever one", as it merely involves a slight inversion of master discourse. Specifically, capitalist discourse inverts the positions between S_1 and $ visible in master discourse.

At this point, it is ready to turn to a diagram of capitalist discourse. Upon close observation, the symbol $ certainly represents the capitalist subject as an agency at the top left. In the diagram, there are S_1 and S_2, which Lacan defines as signifiers. According to Lacan, the signifier is "what represents a subject for another signifier" (Lacan, 1978, p. 51: my translation). Therefore, while the capitalist subject tends to consume itself, it simultaneously represents the agency of capitalist discourse. However, the reality is that this agency is portrayed as another signifier. This implies that the capitalist subject not only is the signifier of agency but also signifies a slave to its own desires. This is why the capitalist subject is denoted as $ in the position of agency; the truth (S_1) of this agency is that it is enslaved by itself. The capitalist subject is no longer the master but rather the other (S_2), which represents a masochistic subject who is willfully castrated and enslaved by their own desires in a capitalist world with no exit. The capitalist subject is trapped within the matrix of the capitalist system due to the *objet a* – surplus-enjoyment, a product of capitalist discourse – located in the top right of the diagram. The capitalist subject becomes addicted to surplus-enjoyment until they find it impossible to exit from a maze of capitalist discourse.

Reflecting on Lacan's capitalist discourse: an anti-structuralist interpretation of capitalist discourse, the Baltimore lecture, and its implications for the proletariat

To fully grasp Lacan's capitalist discourse, it is essential to consider both the concept of the capitalist subject introduced in his Milan speech in 1972 and the imperative discussed in the article "Of Structure as the Inmixing of an Otherness Prerequisite to Any Subject Whatever" (1970). This article is derived from Lacan's lecture in Baltimore in 1966. In his work, Lacan identifies the consumerist subject as a "subject of enjoyment" (*sujet de la jouissance*) (Lacan, 1970 as cited in Macksey and Donato, 2007, p. 195). While the focus is primarily on understanding Lacan's capitalist discourse, it is also important to emphasize the relationship between the consumerist subject and the subject of enjoyment, even though this aspect is not explicitly articulated in Lacan's Milan speech.

In his Baltimore lecture, Lacan discusses the concept of the consumerist subject by presenting a specific example: "Enjoy Coca-Cola" (Lacan, 1970 as cited in Macksey and Donato, 2007, p. 194). His aim is to illustrate the consumerist subject as one driven by enjoyment. A subject of enjoyment refers to an individual who transcends the boundaries set by the pleasure principle, which serves to moderate excessive desire and maintain it at a sufficient level. While capitalism tends to increase the excess of pleasure and enjoyment, the pleasure principle is an inherent psychological mechanism that helps reduce tendencies toward excess. As Lacan stated, "If I am enjoying myself a little too much, I begin to feel pain and I moderate my pleasure" (Lacan, 1970 as cited in Macksey and Donato, 2007, p. 195). The subject of enjoyment – like someone who indulges in

Coca-Cola excessively – shows that capitalism defies this pleasure principle of moderation. This individual is characterized by an unfulfilled desire that persists, aligning them well with capitalist discourse.

Although Lacan's capitalist discourse demonstrates an agreement to disagree with Marx, he does not intend to transcendentalize it, which results in the production of capitalist discourse. In doing so, he seems to undermine and problematize his own discourse. This suggests that anyone overly focused on Lacan's capitalist discourse, who opts to celebrate it as a psychoanalytic critique of capitalism, fails to escape the confines of this discourse and overlooks Lacan's initial warning in his Milan speech. To some extent, it is acceptable for individuals to interpret capitalist discourse by examining the fetishistic relationship between the capitalist subject's lack of profit accumulation and the consumerist subject's lack of desire within a consumption-driven world, mediated by surplus-enjoyment. However, this interpretation reflects a structuralist reading of capitalist discourse. Lacan, in particular, tends to reject interpretations that align his discourse with structuralism. As he stated, "I would not want to join or appear to join this salad called structuralism" (Lacan, 1978, p. 44: my translation). In other words, interpreting Lacan's capitalist discourse through the lens of the structural relationship between the capitalist subject, a masochistic fetishism of the lack, and surplus-enjoyment – considered as an unattainable fulfillment of desire in consumerism – contrasts with Lacan's genuine position and resembles a Copernican scientific approach to his discourse.

The crucial point in Lacan's analysis is that approaching capitalist discourse cannot rely on scientific discourse because "scientific discourse is finalistic, absolutely, in the sense of its functioning" (Lacan, 1978, p. 45: my translation). However, this mechanism of scientific discourse – as a finalistic concept – cannot be separated from its entropic and unconscious aspects. Lacan suggests that scientific discourse, particularly those interpreting capitalist discourse within a structuralist framework, often overlooks an important epistemological rift: the unconscious dimension inherent in capitalist discourse. This oversight allows anyone to push the discourse "towards which brake it is going, and it is necessarily going" (Lacan, 1978, p. 45: my translation). As a result, it is possible to move away from a structuralist interpretation of capitalist discourse, which tends to scholarly repeat a structure of surplus-enjoyment, focusing on the capitalist and consumer subjects within the organizing framework of capitalist production and consumption, while neglecting the potential brakes that could counteract this dynamic.

It is the redundant practice of structuralist interpretation of Lacan's capitalist discourse that leads to the tragedy of being entrapped in capitalism. Therefore, it is largely unjust to hold capitalist and consumerist subjects entirely responsible for ensnaring everyone in this capitalist discourse. Moreover, this structuralist interpretation of capitalist discourse fails to consider Lacan's warning that his discourse represents a transition from closed structures to open structures. As

Lacan states, "I immediately speak of a closed structures and open structures, which is also completely in line with what I am saying now" (Lacan, 1978, p. 44: my translation). In line with Lacan's perspective, capitalist discourse is ultimately untenable because it can shift from a closed system to the open space of self-disruption. This invites contemplation of concepts that differ from the signifier of the capitalist subject, specifically regarding the proletariat.

Ultimately, it is possible to situate the proletariat as a non-relationship within capitalist discourse. When concerns capitalist discourse as a signifier, it presents everyone with what Lacan (1978) describes as "a deceptive signifier" (p. 46: my translation), enticing individuals to concentrate solely on the capitalist subject and the idea of surplus-enjoyment. However, this signifier is "something other than signification" (Lacan, 1978, p. 46: my translation), reflecting the proletariat as the unconscious element within capitalist discourse. It is this unconscious locus that leads to the main thesis of this book: the proletariat discourse, which is linked to four fundamental dimensions: psyche, existence, subject, and politics. These aspects will be elaborated upon in Chapters 2–6.

Exit from the capitalist discourse: 1973–1980

In 1973, one year after his speech in Milan, Lacan engaged in a dialogue with François Cheng, during which he acknowledged Marx's analysis of capitalism and his ability to let it confront its own genuine characteristic. Lacan believed that it was Marx who enabled capitalism to achieve an accurate understanding of its own symptomatic structures. Lacan stated that "it's because of him [Marx] that capitalism has been able to arrive at an accurate analysis of its own structures. In a way, he enabled capitalism to take on its own identity" (Roudinesco, 2005, p. 353). Lacan sought a "way out of capitalist discourse" (Lacan, 1990, p. 16) before it became impossible to restore normalcy. Lacan characterized capitalism as having a "non-sexual relationship" (Lacan, 1990, p. 30), indicating an entropic structure that ultimately brings everything "back to zero" (Lacan, 1990, p. 30) in a severely traumatic manner. However, this does not mean that Lacan politically aligns with the left, which is complacent regarding the possibility of revolution without considering potential contradictions. He suggests that the dogmatic left tends to present itself as virtuous or saintly. Lacan (1990) critiques the misery associated with capitalist discourse (p. 13) and characterizes the leftist "saint" as one who, in reality, "acts as trash" (p. 15).

Following Lacan's caution, a thesis on proletariat discourse asserts that the task of political emancipation from capitalism is one that must be undertaken by the proletariat. However, this discourse aims to avoid complacency and optimism regarding the belief that the proletariat can achieve true revolution without facing internal contradictions, conflicts, or repercussions that might undermine progress. Proletariat discourse does not seek to position itself as infallible or saintly. It intentionally avoids the "pseudo-use of psychoanalysis" (The Žižek

Times, 2025) that Slavoj Žižek has critically cautioned against in contemporary leftist discourse. Proletariat discourse is somewhat linked to leftist ideology; however, it seeks to distinguish itself from the application of Lacanian psychoanalytic concepts to leftist ideology. As the left often fails to adequately address certain gaps, particularly the notion of "the point of the unconscious" (Lacan, 1990, p. 14), this could potentially challenge and overturn the entire discussion put forth by the left. For example, the left's overly optimistic view suggests that the proletariat can assume a position of mastery. However, adopting Lacan's caution signals that within the proletariat lies an unconscious element that, upon revelation, may disrupt their assumed mastery (Lacan, 1990, p. 14).

At this point, despite Lacan addressing Marx's proletariat revolution through the matter of the proletariat as a self-cause, it is advisable to approach the following passage with careful consideration:

> Try not to let go of the handrail regarding what we qua effect of knowledge. Qua effect of knowledge, we are shattered. In the fundamental fantasy ($ <> a) – S barred, lozenge, little a – we are, strange as this may seem, self-caused. And yet, there is no self. Or rather, there is a divided self. The only true political revolution can stem from following this path. Knowledge serves the master. I will return to it again today to highlight that knowledge is born of the slave.
>
> (Lacan, 2024d, p. 341)

In hindsight, Lacan may appear to support Marxist political revolution; however, he thoughtfully explores the limitations and challenges associated with this revolutionary path. As such, it is important to consider three key points that encourage a nuanced interpretation of Lacan's work, particularly to help the left avoid mischaracterizing Lacan as a thinker who entirely aligns with leftist revolutionary ideology: a kind of sainthood.

First, Lacan aims to emphasize a form of knowledge related to the proletariat, which he equates with the position of the slave, but this knowledge is overlooked by the position of the master. His phrases "we are shattered" and "in the fundamental fantasy, we are, strange as this may seem, self-caused" refer to a speculative truth about the proletariat that remains unsymbolized. Although Lacan states that "the slave is left with class consciousness" (Lacan, 2024d, p. 344), the slave or proletariat must be cautious that this class consciousness fails to fulfill a revolutionary mission. Instead, it could be instrumentalized by the party. This perspective often creates a distorted subjective formation for the proletariat, as the party crafts the fantasy that does not convey the true essence of the proletariat (Lacan, 2024e, p. 148).

Second, Lacan's expression of "self-caused" encourages the proletariat to philosophically and psychoanalytically examine their own subjectivities. This inquiry may lead to a speculative, though not absolute, understanding of themselves. If the absolutization of truth is impossible, then the proletariat will similarly struggle to achieve an absolute understanding of their own existence. Lacan contends that the pursuit of truth as a form of absolutization is an idealistic endeavor. He asserts that "if truth is not knowledge, then it is non-knowledge. That's Aristotelian logic – everything that is not black is non-black" (Lacan, 2017, p. 10). This suggests that anything that is not black cannot be fully captured as absolute knowledge, as there remains an unwritten aspect of the non-black that exists outside the realm of absolute knowledge. As a result, attempts to articulate this often fall short.

By highlighting the connection between Lacan and the proletariat that arises from political revolution, one can see a reflection of the left's political optimism. This viewpoint aims to integrate psychoanalysis into political discourse, though it sometimes does so with insufficient caution. Lacan's phrase "self-caused" serves as a warning for the proletariat: they may also encounter "the symptom", or a gap within their own cause, which reveals their own genuine "truth-value" (p. 45). This realization prompts the proletariat to reconsider their subjectivities beyond the party's exploitation of their class consciousness for its own political interest. As noted by Chris Vanderwees (2019),

> Lacan does not refer to any sort of universalization or institutionalization of truth, but rather to the singular truth of each subject, a form of knowledge that emerges in the subject's relation to the symbolic that emerges at the point of its lack.
>
> (p. 105)

This indicates that the proletariat, as "self-caused", can be understood as a political agent for revolution. However, they must also remain aware of any gaps or deficiencies present within their own experience, as they may encounter what Lacan describes as "knowledge that is not known to the subject" (Lacan, 2024d, p. 348).

Third, Lacan expresses concern that the proletariat may find themselves in a situation where they experience both a "divided self" and a "no self". The term "no self" does not imply the inexistence of the proletariat. Instead, it suggests that the concepts of a divided self and a "no self" – knowledge that is outside the symbolic order – could persist even in a post-capitalist and extensively a communist world. In this sense, following Lacan's insight, this particular type of proletariat could recognize a void in their own subjectivity and transform into something unfamiliar to Marx. This transformation might evoke a sense of uncanniness for Marx. It is insufficient to simply state that a communist haunts capitalist society but rather a proletariat that could haunt its own communist world. Ultimately, it could destabilize a communist society, propelled by the actions of the proletariat themselves.

The three points mentioned earlier serve as a modest cautionary note to left-wing ideologists who engage with Lacanian psychoanalysis in their pursuit of revolutionary politics. Nevertheless, in 1980, during his declaration of the Dissolution of Psychoanalysis, Lacan – who passed away a year later – offered his insights on the concept of the proletariat in the following manner:

> I paid homage to Marx as the inventor of the symptom. This Marx is, however, the restorer of order, simply because he has reinspired among the proletariat the *dit-mension* (di-mention/mention of the said) of meaning. For that, it was enough for the proletariat to say it.
>
> (Lacan as cited in Lippi, p. 184)

Upon reflection, this passage should be approached with caution. It does not imply that Lacan aligns himself with communist ideology, advocating for a classless society or endorsing a linear view of history. While the proletariat is presented in this passage as a historical truth, one should be careful to avoid any tendency toward complacency in this interpretation.

The passage can be divided into two main points. First, Lacan regards Marx as the "inventor of the symptom" within capitalist discourse, allowing the capitalist system to confront its true face. Second, Lacan perceives that Marx has "reinspired among the proletariat the *dit-mension* (di-mention/mention of the said) of meaning". This perspective suggests that the proletariat is destined to be "the restorer of order" – a liberator from capitalism – and that is the end of it: "it was enough for the proletariat to say it". However, such a teleological viewpoint is overly optimistic. The crucial aspect of this discussion lies in the term *dit-mension* used in this context, which implies that meaning encompasses more than what is explicitly stated. According to Sylvia Lippi, Lacan's concept of *dit-mension* refers to "the remaining forgotten and behind what is said in what is heard" (Lacan as cited in Lippi, 2022, p. 186). This notion operates in conjunction with considerations of the unconscious and the inherent gaps within the proletariat itself.

To avoid becoming rigid and forming an overly dogmatic sainthood, proletariat discourse must not ignore the inherent gaps and shortcomings within the proletariat itself. Lacan explains that the unconscious represents this gap. He uses the metaphor of "alternating suction" to illustrate that the unconscious is a place for genuine radical thought, which is often forgotten or overlooked. It is from this space that thoughts emerge, allowing one to hear things that may have otherwise been disregarded because they were not properly recognized (Lacan, 2006b, pp. 710–711). Furthermore, the term *dire* in Lacan's concept of *dit-mension* relates to something that is articulated and seeks to establish itself as absolute knowledge, such as "the restorer of order". However, this desire is hindered by the symptoms and ontological incompleteness present in the unconscious, preventing the attainment of such a status. Lacan's caution serves to guide the speculative truth of the proletariat incorporated in proletariat discourse, away from the uncritical application of Lacanian psychoanalysis in political contexts by the contemporary left.

To sum up this chapter, Lacan's concept of capitalist discourse is situated within the framework of psychoanalytic discourse. He engages with Marx's analysis of the proletariat through the lens of surplus-value, based on his idea of surplus-enjoyment. However, Lacan cautions against interpreting capitalist discourse solely through a structuralist approach, highlighting that capitalist discourse is rather a sliding signifier, indicating the position of the proletariat. Eventually, the proletariat discourse says to capitalist discourse, "You never look at me from the place I see you". Capitalist discourse is in the proletariat's gaze, but proletariat is not pictured clearly in the capitalist discourse. While it is essential to exit capitalist discourse by depending on the proletariat, Lacan warns that the ontological deficiency of the proletariat could disrupt the teleological narrative of the revolutionary process.

Reference list

Alemán, J. (2024). *Lacan and Capitalist Discourse: Neoliberalism and Ideology*. New York and Oxon: Routledge.

Bianchi, P. (2010). 'The Discourse and the Capitalist: Lacan, Marx, and the Questions of the Surplus', *Folozofski vestnik,* XXXI(2), 123–137.

Bruno, P. (2020). *Lacan and Marx: The Invention of the Symptom*. Translated by John Holland. New York and Oxon: Routledge.

Freud, S. (2010). 'Consciousness and the Unconscious', in *The Ego and the Id*. New York: Pacific Publishing Studio.

Lacan, J. (1966a). Unpublished text. *The Seminar of Jacques Lacan Book XIII: The Object of Psychoanalysis*. English translation is from an unpublished text by Cormac Gallagher. Available at: http://www.lacaninireland.com/web/wp-content/uploads/2010/06/13-The-Object-of-Psychoanalysis1.pdf. Accessed: April 5, 2025.

Lacan, J. (1966b). Unpublished text. *The Seminar of Jacques Lacan Book XIV: The Logic of Phantasy*. English translation is from an unpublished text by Cormac Gallagher. Available at: http://www.lacaninireland.com/web/wp-content/uploads/2010/06/THE-SEMINAR-OF-JACQUES-LACAN-XIV.pdf. Accessed: April 5, 2025.

Lacan, J. (1970). 'Of structure as an Inmixing of an Otherness Prerequisite to Any Subject Whatever', in *The Structuralist Controversy: The Language of Criticism and the Sciences of Man*. Edited by R. Macksey, and E. Donato. 40th Anniversary Edition. Baltimore: The John Hopkins University Press.

Lacan, J. (1973). 'Italian Note'. English translation is from an unpublished text by Cormac Gallagher. Available at: https://www.lacaninireland.com/wp-content/uploads/2010/06/Italian-note-1973.pdf. Accessed: January 30, 2026.

Lacan, J. (1978). 'Discours de Jacques Lacan à l'Université de Milan le 12 mai 1972, paru dans l'ouvrage bilingue': Lacan in Italia 1953–1978. En Italie Lacan, Milan, *La Salamandra*: pp. 32–55.

Lacan, J. (1981a). 'Alienation', in *The Seminar of Jacques Lacan Book XI: The Four Fundamental Concepts of Psychoanalysis*. Edited by Jacques-Alain Miller. Translated by Alan Sheridan. London and New York: W.W. Norton Company.

Lacan, J. (1981b). 'The Line and Light', in *The Seminar of Jacques Lacan Book XI: The Four Fundamental Concepts of Psychoanalysis*. Edited by Jacques-Alain Miller. Translated by Alan Sheridan. London and New York: W.W. Norton Company.

Lacan, J. (1990). *Jacques Lacan Television: A Challenge to the Psychoanalytic Establishment*. Translated by Jeffrey Mehlman. London and New York: W.W. Norton & Company.
Lacan, J. (2006a). 'Kant with Sade', in *Écrits: The First Complete Edition in English*. Translated by Bruce Fink. London and New York: W.W. Norton & Company.
Lacan, J. (2006b). 'Position of the Unconscious', in *Écrits: The First Complete Edition in English*. Translated by Bruce Fink. London and New York: W.W. Norton & Company.
Lacan, J. (2006c). 'Science and Truth', in *Écrits: The First Complete Edition in English*. Translated by Bruce Fink. London and New York: W.W. Norton & Company.
Lacan, J. (2006d). 'The Freudian Thing or the Meaning of the Return to Freud in Psychoanalysis', in *Écrits: The First Complete Edition in English*. Translated by Bruce Fink. London and New York: W.W. Norton & Company.
Lacan, J. (2008a). 'The Death Drive', in *The Seminar of Jacques Lacan Book VII: The Ethics of Psychoanalysis*. Translated by Dennis Porter. Oxon and New York: Routledge.
Lacan, J. (2008b). 'The Object and the Thing', in *The Seminar of Jacques Lacan Book VII: The Ethics of Psychoanalysis*. Translated by Dennis Porter. Oxon and New York: Routledge.
Lacan, J. (2017). *Talking to Brick Walls: A Series of Presentations in the Chapel at the Sainte-Anne Hospital*. Translated by Adrian Price. Cambridge: Polity Press.
Lacan, J. (2024a). 'From Surplus Value to Surplus Jouissance', in *The Seminar of Jacques Lacan: Book XVI: From an Other to the Other*. Translated by Bruce Fink. Cambridge and New Jersey: Polity Press.
Lacan, J. (2024b). 'Paradoxes of Psychoanalytic Action', in *The Seminar of Jacques Lacan: Book XVI: From an Other to the Other*. Translated by Bruce Fink. Cambridge and New Jersey: Polity Press.
Lacan, J. (2024c). 'The Knowledge Market and Truth (On) Strike', in *The Seminar of Jacques Lacan: Book XVI: From an Other to the Other*. Translated by Bruce Fink. Cambridge and New Jersey: Polity Press.
Lacan, J. (2024d). 'The Ravishing Ignominy of the *Hommelle*', in *The Seminar of Jacques Lacan: Book XVI: From an Other to the Other*. Translated by Bruce Fink. Cambridge and New Jersey: Polity Press.
Lacan, J. (2024e). 'Truth's Retardation and the Administration of Knowledge', in *The Seminar of Jacques Lacan: Book XVI: From an Other to the Other*. Translated by Bruce Fink. Cambridge and New Jersey: Polity Press.
Lee, M. (2022). 'Perversion After Freud: From the Cruel Father to the Joycean Clinic', in *Lacan's Cruelty: Perversion beyond Philosophy, Culture and Clinic*. Edited by M. Lee. Cham: Palgrave Macmillan.
Lippi, Silvia S. (2022). '"Proletarian/labourer/worker"', in *The Marx Through Lacan Vocabulary: A Compass for Libidinal and Political Economies*. Edited by Christina Soto van der Plas, Edgar Miguel Juárez-Salazar, and Carlos Gómez Camarena. Oxon and New York: Routledge
Moncayo, R., Belnap, B., and Farr, G. (2024). *Exploring Lacan's Encore Seminar XX: The Torus of Reason*. Oxon and New York: Routledge.
Roudinesco, E. (2005). *Jacques Lacan: An Outline of a Life and a History of a System of Thought*. Translated by Barbara Bray. New York: Columbia University Press.
Swales, S. (2022). 'Neoliberalism and Liminality: Perverse Cruelties in the Age of Capitalist Discourse', in *Lacan's Cruelty: Perversion beyond Philosophy, Culture and Clinic*. Edited by M. Lee. Cham: Palgrave Macmillan.
Tomšič, S. (2019). *The Labour of Enjoyment: Towards a Critique of Libidinal Economy*. Berlin: August Verlag.
Tomšič, Samo. (2015). *The Capitalist Unconscious: Marx and Lacan*. London and New York: Verso.

Vanderwees, C. (2019). 'Jacques Lacan Talking to Brick Walls: A Series of Presentations in the Chapel at the Saint-Anne Hospital. Translated by A. R. Price'. *Psychoanalytic Discourse*, 4(1), 104–108.

Vanheule, S. (2016). 'Capitalist Discourse, Subjectivity, and Lacanian Psychoanalysis', *Frontiers in Psychology*, (7), 1–15. doi: https://doi.org/10.3389/fpsyg.2016.01948. Accessed: May 14, 2025.

Zevnik, A. (2022). 'Capitalism', in *The Marx Through Lacan Vocabulary: A Compass for Libidinal and Political Economies*. Edited by Christina Soto van der Plas, Edgar Miguel Juárez-Salazar, and Carlos Gómez Camarena. Oxon and New York: Routledge.

Žižek, S. (2025). 'Slavoj Žižek: I'm against pseudo use of psychoanalysis', *The Žižek Times*. April 27. 22.52 mins. Available at https://www.youtube.com/watch?v=FBIxdXP2zPc. Accessed: May 11, 2025.

3 Hysterical proletariat and the specter of communism

From the specter of Marx to the specter that haunts Marx

This chapter aims to reinterpret Karl Marx's concept of the proletariat, which is characterized as the "spectre of communism" (Marx and Engels, 2004, p. 19) – communism serves as a new power of opposition to the old power of capitalism and reflects a human being whose unpleasant, exploited, expropriated, and dispossessed life illustrates an ontological dissonance within the pleasure principle of capitalism – through Jacques Lacan's psychoanalytical view of the hysteric. Marx's specter of communism resembles Lacan's concept of the hysteric, particularly in the context of Lacan's hysteric discourse. The thesis of the proletariat discourse posits that Lacan's concept of the hysteric allows for the existence of a hysterical proletariat. This hysterical proletariat shares certain characteristics with Marx's proletariat, but it also represents an entity that transcends Marx's original imagination. While capitalism reflects the reality of social relations and is haunted by Marx's specter – a revival of his ideology championed by the Left advocating for social change – it is the psychoanalytic hysterical proletariat that emerges as a potential entity haunting Marx himself.

To reemphasize, this chapter addresses the relationship and the gap between Lacan's notion of the hysteric and Marx's idea of the specter of communism. The analysis presents the emergence of what this chapter identifies as the hysterical proletariat, which is understood through four fundamental dimensions of proletariat discourse: psyche, existence, subject, and politics. The arguments are organized into four main sections. The first section discusses the psyche of the hysteric, highlighting its connection to the psychoanalytic concept of aphasia: a discrepancy exists between the subject's inner desire and how that desire is expressed to the outside world. This leads to an exploration of the gap between Marx's understanding of the proletariat and the portrayal of the proletariat as representing aphasia. The second section focuses on hysterical existence, depicting the proletariat as a hysteric who desires a master, yet the master fails to control them. This perspective brings to light a psychoanalytic aspect that Marx may not fully address in his analysis of the proletariat. In the third section, the discussion shifts to the hysterical subject. Here, the proletariat is seen as a hysteric

DOI: 10.4324/9781003657781-3

who seeks to conquer the communist ideal but ultimately finds dissatisfaction with it. This creates a gap between Marx's vision of communism and the proletariat's idealization of communism, which may not fully align with Marx's initial principles. The final section addresses the proletariat's universal politics of anti-capitalism as the sublime hysteric. This concept suggests that the proletariat's resistance to capitalism aims to achieve a deeper, speculative understanding and truth about itself.

A hysterical psyche: a revision of Freud's hysteric, the aphasia, and Marx's proletariat

To understand the emergence of the hysterical psyche, it is necessary to highlight that the psyche is not a unified self; rather, it is a dialectically self-divided entity. The influence of Hegelian dialectics leads Lacan to reinterpret Sigmund Freud's Gestalt of the hysteric. Freud and Joseph Breuer characterize hysterics as individuals with mental disorders. In a clinical setting, they scientifically identify the hysteric as someone who has a fixed object of desire – an object associated with past unfulfillment. The repression surrounding this fixation compels the subject to repeatedly engage with this unfulfilled desire. Freud's insights into the hysterical psyche are detailed in *Studies in Hysteria* (1895), one of his important works from the pre-psychoanalytic period. This publication could be regarded as a prelude to Freud's official introduction of "psychoanalysis" as a medical field a year later, in 1896, when he was 40 years old.

In Freud's pre-psychoanalytic understanding of the hysteric's psyche, its Gestalt reveals the presence of a hidden memory. This hidden memory not only indicates a secret that the hysterical individual conceals but also suggests the origin of trauma. The origin of trauma is something that the hysterical individual cannot control, as it is driven by the forces of the unconscious that continually resurface beyond the individual's conscious awareness. Freud describes the unconscious as consisting of "thoughts that did not materialize" (Freud and Breuer, 2024, p. 301). It is within the unconscious that the true psyche of the hysteric can be found. Thus, understanding the hysteric's psyche requires the psychoanalyst to recognize the presence of hysterical suffering and to identify with "the existence of hidden, unconscious motives" (Freud and Breuer, 2024, p. 295). This psychoanalytic method aims to access the hysteric's inner world. Freud elaborates on this in the following text.

> When I have promised my patients help or relief by means of a cathartic treatment, I have repeatedly had to listen to the following objection: 'You yourself tell me that what I am suffering from is probably connected with my circumstances and fate. You can't change anything about that. So how are you going to help me?' And I have been able to answer: 'I do not doubt that it would be easier for fate to take away your suffering than it would for me. But you

> will see for yourself that much has been gained if we succeed in turning your hysterical misery into common unhappiness. Having restored your inner life, you will be better able to arm yourself against that unhappiness.
>
> (Freud and Breuer, 2024, p. 306)

According to the passage, a fundamental issue in Freud's understanding of hysteric is that he sees the hysterical psyche as being shaped by a lack of sexual gratification. A hysteric is characterized by feelings of sexual dissatisfaction, and Freud's notion of hysterical misery suggests a unity of self within the hysteric. Hysterical misery results from the inhibition of desire, which leads to a configuration of unconscious motives. Freud's approach to hysteric is clinically limited to a purely analytic technique. Freud's patients often experience mental depression, and through therapy, they come to understand that their suffering and psychological issues are influenced by fate. This concept of fate can manifest in various ways, such as through God, a transcendental entity, or past karma in certain cultures and religions. In an attempt to console his patients, Freud suggests that they transform their "hysterical misery into common unhappiness". This suggestion does not indicate Freud's political ideologies but rather suggests that it is normal for everyone to experience hysterical misery and to be influenced by civilization in relation to collective dissatisfaction. Lacan also reacts positively to Freud's *Studies of Hysteria*. Lacan states,

> I only have to remind you of the *Studien über Hysterie*, which is nothing other than one long account of the discovery of the analytic technique. That is where we witness it in the making, and this is what makes these studies priceless.
>
> (Lacan, 1991, p. 9)

Lacan's reinterpretation of the hysteric differs significantly from Freud's original perspective. The process begins with a sense of lack – the unfulfillment of desire – which is stored in the unconscious. It is this lack that develops into the object of desire to which the hysteric is related. Lacan presents hysteric as a representation of the psychoanalytic subject that expresses internalized repressive desires without seeking reconciliation with the social norms that enforce prohibition. The repressive desires developed by the unconscious are what the hysteric as the "subject has to take possession of it" (Lacan, 1986b, p. 72). The hysteric is an unconventional way of living that transgresses these prohibitions and the repressive social order, having the potential to disrupt an entire civilization. Importantly, the hysteric is not confined to clinical settings or to individuals with mental disturbances; this form of hysterical subjectivity is the realist subject that is impossible for the symbolic order (Fierens, 2022) but exists in everyone to varying degrees. Thus, the hysteric illustrates an individual's rejection of self-certainty and a preservation of desire without yielding to social conventions.

The hysteric embodies the Real; this way of being is neither the ideal ego (the self is aligned with a pre-linguistic stage) nor the ego-ideal (the self that adheres to the desires of the Other within a linguistic framework) (Lacan, 1986a, p. 49).

Lacan effectively moves beyond Freud's concept of the hysterical psyche, which is limited to a clinical setting. In Lacan's view, the hysteric represents the Real, highlighting that the ego is an essential component. The ego serves as a foundation for the subject to reflect on symptoms in relation to the desire of the Other, which the subject ultimately must negate. In other words, a hysterical psyche strives to deny the concept of *res cognitas*. This notion indicates that consciousness is shaped by the desires of the Other. Negating *res cognitas* does not imply that the Other is absent or completely dismissed. Rather, it signifies the need to maintain a space where the hysteric, as the Real, can contemplate and seek a genuine sense of belonging (Lacan, 1986a, p. 49).

This highlights the fundamental nature of the hysterical psyche, emphasizing its movement from the ideal state of emptiness to a more materialistic perspective. In a pre-linguistic phase, the psyche exists merely as an empty vessel, only to be shaped by external influences. Once this shaping occurs, the psyche begins to form through the reliance on language. A key principle of the psyche is that it is not driven by instinct; instead, it requires the invention of language to function and think. This principle suggests that the psyche acts as a mirror reflecting language. The influence of language on the psyche generates a form of idealism that can lead to a disconnection from the psyche's true essence. This alienation results in a sort of paralysis within the psyche itself. Specifically, the hysterical psyche experiences an urgent desire to communicate its experience of lack that unconscious never lets it go (Lichtenstein, 2018). Ultimately, as the sublime of the clinical, social, and political voice, the hysterical desire evolves into a need for its speech to manifest as an action that seeks to affirm its own speculative truth.

Demanding a new master but receiving the aphasic one

There is a commonly held interpretation of Lacan's notion of the hysteric that evolves into a hypothesis *ad infinitum*, forming a general understanding of Lacan's concept. This hypothesis posits that the hysteric demands a new master, only to discover that they receive not a better leader, but a repressive one – often deemed worse than the previous master. This understanding stems from Lacan's response to the student protests at the Experimental University in Vincennes on December 3, 1969. On that day, Lacan addressed the students' disruptive interference with his teaching in the following manner:

> *INTERVENTION:* One could say that Lenin almost became aphasic.
>
> [Lacan:] If you had a bit of patience, and if you really wanted our impromptus to continue, I would tell you that, always, the revolutionary aspiration has

> only a single possible outcome – of ending up as the master's discourse. This is what experience has proved.
>
> What you aspire to as revolutionaries is a master. You will get one.
>
> (Lacan, 2007a, p. 207)

There are two significant observations regarding the original source quoted earlier. First and foremost, the term "hysteric" does not actually appear in the original text. This raises some important questions about the hypothesis suggesting that Lacan identifies the rebellious students as the revolutionary hysteric demanding a new master – one who may ultimately be even worse than the current one. Second, what remains ambiguous and somewhat lacking in the quote derived from the original texts is the new master's tendency toward an oppressive regime, a regime that would impede the genuine social change the revolutionaries seek. It is important to approach this understanding of the hysteric with caution. It may be useful but ultimately inconclusive. Lacan's quick response to those questioning his teachings was just that – a brief, one-off reply given during a specific moment, which does not fully encapsulate his theory on the hysteric. This is especially significant considering that Lacan was not entirely in control of his faculties at the time.

Instead, the passage suggests that the discussion between Lacan and the student centers on Lenin's tendency toward aphasia, which should be regarded as a primary focus. Unfortunately, the concept of aphasia does not receive much attention in the works of Lacanian scholars. However, when approached thoughtfully, this concept aligns well with Lacan's understanding of discourse and is a valuable psychoanalytic idea.

In essence, aphasia refers to the element that disrupts social connections. Lacan explains aphasia as follows: "just think that there are people who happen to have things in their brain and who no longer have any idea how to manage with language. That makes them somewhat crippled" (Lacan, 2007a, p. 207). If the function of discourse is to forge social bonds, then aphasia serves as a plague or an impossibility within that discourse. Understanding aphasia is crucial for grasping Lacan's critique of discourse as a social bond. It underscores the gap between a person's true self or thoughts and their lack of expression of those thoughts clearly and completely by depending on language. This gap between a subject's true thinking and their linguistic expression can occur in anyone, not just in the psychotic or the neurotic. In this discussion, Lenin is depicted as a master revolutionary who establishes an authoritarian regime. However, a conversation between Lacan and a student focuses on Lenin's potential experience of aphasia, which creates a divide between his true being or true thinking and his discursive communication to the public. This gap between truth and language results in a rupture of the political relationship between the sovereign and the subject. Eventually, what is intended to be a political administration becomes unmanageable, leading to a disorderly political order.

In short, regarding the understanding of the hysteric and the aphasic, it is insufficient to simply reference a general notion that the hysteric seeks a new master. This new master is likely to be oppressive, potentially even worse than the previous one. A more nuanced argument should emphasize that while the hysteric demands a new master, they often receive an aphasic one, a scenario that is likely common in various political regimes. Regardless of whether this new master is authoritarian, it is important to note that the master sought by the hysteric will often resemble the old master. This creates a situation in which meaningful political change is unlikely, as the new master could exhibit aphasia. Consequently, there is often a disconnect between the sovereign's true intentions and their expression in language, and this issue can also arise within democratic systems.

A proletariat psyche as aphasic: a thinking being and a materialism of the hysterical psyche

A proletariat psyche can be understood as aphasic, representing a thinking being and a materialism rooted in a hysterical psyche. The concept of a hysterical psyche, which has the potential to be aphasic, can be used to explore the psyche of the proletariat. This perspective goes beyond Marxism's reduction of the proletariat to mere class consciousness. The hysterical psyche introduces an element of uncanniness to Marx's understanding of the proletariat, as he tends to overlook this dimension.

Based on the existing context of aphasia mentioned earlier and in relation to Lacan's psychoanalytic concepts, Marx's concept of the proletariat should not be equated with a psychotic individual or a madman. There is a complex aspect to the proletariat's psyche. Similar to Lenin, in a discussion between Lacan and an uprising student, and by revisiting this issue within the same framework, it can be argued that Marx's proletariat creates a distinction between the proletariat as a being engaged in language – being-in-language – and the proletariat as a thinking being.

If this is the case, what is the potential aphasia of Marx's proletariat? It reflects a symptom related to the communist world, which serves as an object of desire, highlighting a gap between the proletariat as a being-in-language according to Marx and the proletariat's true communist world as a thinking being. This gap arises because Marx's imagination of communism for the proletariat is ultimately flawed and incomplete, revealing an inherent aphasia:

1. Abolition of the property in land and application of all rents of land to public purposes
2. A heavy progressive or graduated income tax
3. Abolition of all right of inheritance

4. Confiscation of the property of all emigrants and rebels
5. Centralization of credit in the hands of the State, by means of a national bank with State capital and an exclusive monopoly
6. Centralization of the means of communication and transport in the hands of the State
7. Extension of factories and instruments of production owned by the State; the bringing into cultivation of waste-lands, and the improvement of the soil generally in accordance with a common plan
8. Equal liability of all to labor. Establishment of industrial armies, especially for agriculture
9. Combination of agriculture with manufacturing industries; gradual abolition of the distinction between town and country, by a more equable distribution of the population over the country.
10. Free education for all children in public schools. Abolition of children's factory labor in its present form. Combination of education with industrial production, &c., &c.

(Marx and Engels, 2004, p. 48)

The philosophical significance of the proletariat's complex psyche begins with a fundamental question: is the communist imaginary envisioned by Marx fully accepted by the proletariat? If it is accepted, does this indicate a sense of incompleteness? By exploring the concept of aphasia, one can gain a better understanding of the gap between the proletariat's perspective of communism as their true existence and the image of communism articulated by Marx's language. The concept of aphasia suggests that the authentic thoughts of the proletariat regarding the communist world may include elements that are inexplicable and cannot be fully expressed in words like those of Marx. This implies a substantial gap in the proletariat's understanding, which exists between Marx's depiction of the communist imaginary and a deeper truth that transcends Marx's existing conceptual framework.

This situation goes beyond simply viewing the proletariat through the lens of class consciousness. The central issue is whether the proletariat and their visions of a communist world can be shaped by Marx's deterministic and formative language. In response, it is likely that the realm of the proletariat's hysterical psyche will give rise to the communist imagination, which is different from Marx's initial imagination. Thus, this expression can be counterproductive to Marx, resembling a "solid that has melted into air" due to the theoretical constraints he imposes. This observation suggests a potential limitation in Marx's work, as he may not have fully recognized the significance of the hysterical psyche and aphasia. In reality, when the proletariat experiences a hysterical psyche, it allows them to envision a communist imaginary from a different perspective. If Marx's portrayal of the communist imaginary embodies self-certainty, then it might suggest that the guidance he provides to the proletariat could benefit from further exploration to address any ontological incompleteness.

At this point, a Hegelian positive negation from the perspective of the hysterical psyche of the proletariat has become a philosophical necessity. For this psyche, it is Hegel who serves as a critique of Marx, rather than Marx critiquing Hegel. In other words, for the hysterical proletariat, Hegel is seen as a dialectical materialist philosopher closely aligned with Lacan, who introduces a symptom to Marx's theories, culminating in the creation of a symptom for Marx's vision of communism. This highlights the materialism inherent in the hysterical psyche of the proletariat. This concept suggests that when one considers the hysterical proletariat and its ontological psyche, the issue arises from a hypothesis centered around the subordination of the psyche to the distorting language present in Marx's representation of the communist ideal. In Lacanian terms, this reflects a lack within the psyche that has been ontologically erased by a form of knowledge rooted in Marx's manifesto. In response, there is an act of sublation of the psyche, which transforms it into a compelling and substantial radical substance. As a result, the essence of the psyche – specifically that of the hysterical proletariat – must reemerge and reposition itself as a truth in opposition to this knowledge. This process must take place in a manner that diverges from conventional discourse and the limitations of language.

Hegel's philosophy significantly influences Lacan's understanding of the hysterical psyche. To grasp the hysterical psyche fully, it is essential to consider both the role of language and the concept of repressed desire. In Hegel's philosophy, language serves as both a ground of being and a ground of negativity, suggesting that language reveals absolute abstraction. When stating that language is a ground of being, it is acknowledged that language shapes the material nature of the void. Language ultimately leads to the creation of an ideal image of the subject's psyche. This ideal image represents the void – the very first essence of the void – since it embodies a form of absolute idealism. This idea aligns with Hegel's "two propositions" discussed in *Science of Logic*. These propositions relate to Hegel's thoughts on the concept of essence, which he asserts must manifest: "essence must appear" (Hegel, 2010a, p. 418).

In the first proposition, Hegel states that "the doctrine of being contains the first proposition, 'being is essence'" (Hegel, 2010a, p. 418). From a Lacanian perspective, this initial proposition of Hegel represents the psyche as a product of the structural reality determined by language. However, this psyche does not reveal the truth of the self; it is merely a semblance of the psyche – representing a lack or less than what is supposed to be [*en deçà*] (Lacan, 2006a, p. 40). In the relationship between Hegel and Lacan, it is inevitable that the subject's psyche is shaped by language. This creates a paradox where the psyche is summoned by language in order to be integrated into it. Marx's manifesto represents the image of communism as a ground of being. Nevertheless, this ontological gap, which is identified by both Hegel and Lacan, serves as a foundation for negation. When the ideal image of the subject's psyche is transformed into a material subject, this material subject's psyche begins to critique the very ground of language that summoned it. The psyche, now materialized and even more radicalized, undergoes the process of self-sublation. During this process, the ideal image of the subject's psyche – previously confined within the domain of language – begins to negate itself by emphasizing a voice of its own, ultimately resulting in the psyche of the hysterical subject as the material subject. However, the material psyche is not an endpoint. A vacuum or gap persists within the psyche, which the subject is compelled to confront.

In the second proposition, Hegel states that "essence is being". This notion highlights that the essence of being emerges through negativity and a critical inward reflection on language, order, and a dominant public consciousness. According to Hegel, this proposition refers to an essence of being, which can be described as "concrete existence [*die Existenz*], a being that has emerged from negativity and inwardness" (Hegel, 2010a, p. 418). The concrete existence is the unity that contains a dimension of thought that compels the unity to externalize itself from its existential unity (Hegel, 2010b, p. 154). This idea aligns with Lacan's acknowledgment of a deprivation of the stability of the symbolic language. It stems from the concept of lack, leading to the quest for the possible essence of being. The material aspect of the psyche is dialectical; it must break free from the constraints of language that overdetermine it. However, when the psyche successfully transforms into a blend of positive and negative qualities, moving beyond the constraints of language, this inwardness can be viewed as a form of materialism. This state of being represents a foundation of negation, in which the speculative truth of the proletariat's communism diverges from the communist ideal Marx envisioned for them. This complex hysterical psyche of the proletariat finds reconciliation within this Hegelian essence.

A hysterical existence: the proletariat and a master who fails to reign

In this section, the term "existence" refers to the hysteric's inquiry and interpretation of their surrounding situation. This process allows the hysteric to separate from their environment and eventually embrace an extraordinary lifestyle. The existence of the hysteric inspires a discourse framing the proletariat's condition as hysterical. This concept was observed on April 8, 1970. Unlike the discussions at Vincennes in 1969, Lacan was fully aware during this presentation and was not interrupted by students. Lacan challenged his audience with the question: "What does the hysteric want?" Lacan responded, stating that "she wants a master". According to Lacan, for the hysteric, "she wants the other to be a master, and to know lots of things" (Lacan, 2007b, p. 129). Nonetheless, he continues that, significantly,

> but at the same time she doesn't want him to know so much that he does not believe she is the supreme price of all his knowledge. In other words, she wants a master she can reign over. She reigns, and he does not govern.
>
> (Lacan, 2007b, p. 129)

The existence of the hysteric represents a desire for power and control. The hysteric seeks a master, but paradoxically, this master must be one who fails to exercise complete authority. While a master may govern the hysteric, the hysteric's desire remains elusive to the master. The hysteric's desire is akin to the concept of the *objet a*, which signifies a non-relationship that is inherent in every discourse but often goes unnoticed. Lacan illustrates a gap between the true essence of the hysteric, which remains mysterious to the master, and the master's limited understanding of the hysteric's thoughts. Consequently, this discrepancy results in a symptom and creates tension within the socio-political relationships. The desire of the hysteric indicates the decline of the master. The hysteric challenges and disrupts the social order established by the master. The master represents the narratives and historical accounts that highlight a symptomatic void – the existence of the hysteric – that these accounts fail to include (Žižek, 2014, p. 74).

In terms of existence, the hysteric pays a "supreme price" that transcends the master's possession of knowledge about her. The hysteric desires a master who ultimately fails to govern her, as her true aim is not to have a master but to dominate the master instead. Consequently, the master is nearly reduced to the level of non-existence. It is a misconception to view the relationship between the hysteric and the master as transcendental. This misunderstanding encourages an exploration of the conflict between the discourse of the master and the discourse of the hysteric. The concept of the symptom defines an inherently impossible relationship between the master and the hysteric. This reality explains why hysterical existence is resistant to conforming with the master. Instead, it seeks to distance itself from the master, pursuing its own distinct style of life, as Lacan elucidates that "at the level of the hysteric's discourse it is clear that we see this dominant appears in the form of a symptom. It is around the symptom that the hysteric's discourse is situated and ordered" (Lacan, 2007d, p. 43).

Hysterical existence shows that its desire either illuminates the unsignified or emphasizes the mysterious signifier for the master; in this case, the sovereign is blinded to such a mystical signifier. This situation reflects an ontological discordance between the master's knowledge of the hysteric and the hysteric's desire, which remains enigmatic and unsignified. While the hysteric does not become a master herself, her latent desire does not completely construct a metaphysical knowledge for the master. This is why the master repeatedly fails and undermines his own authority. The incommensurability between the master and the hysteric can be observed across different political systems, including democracy, socialism, and Marx's vision of communism. In this context, the disruptive conditions of a communist ideal may arise from the hysterical existence of the proletariat. This insight, derived from a psychoanalytic perspective, serves as a cautionary reminder to Marx and traditional Marxism.

Proletariat as hysterical existence: encountering a master who fails to reign

To understand the proletariat as a hysterical existence, Lacan introduces the term "existence" (*ex-sistence*) to denote something that questions and separates itself from its existing surroundings, as noted in the introductory chapter. By integrating Lacan's insights with those of Marx, common ground can be identified between the two thinkers. Marx encourages the proletariat to critically examine and distance themselves from the prevailing capitalist conditions, which, in his time, included factories, and in the present, extend to digital platforms. However, the most significant aspect is that psychoanalysis rather serves as a critical inquiry into the limitations of Marxism, addressing elements of thought that Marxism often overlooks. The purpose of a psychoanalytic intervention, which symbolizes the invention of the symptom for Marx, is not to act as a counter-revolution but rather to encourage Marxism to develop and refine its own existing theories. This is how Lacanian psychoanalysis is valuable and fosters a constructive dialogue with Marx's theories on anti-capitalism and the proletariat. In this context, it is insufficient to simply claim that Marx is the inventor of the symptom related to capitalism. Rather, Marx's perspective on the proletariat neglects a crucial psychoanalytic dimension – the hysterical existence of the proletariat. It is this specter of the proletariat that symbolizes a specter that haunts Marx.

Essentially, this implies that upon revisiting Marx's concept of "the specter of communism" related to the proletariat as articulated in *The Communist Manifesto*, a psychoanalytic perspective, particularly one informed by Lacan, suggests that Marx's assertion that "a specter is haunting Europe – the specter of communism" (Marx and Engels, 2004, p. 19) is insufficient. According to Lacan, the hysteric embodies a "supreme price", indicating that the hysteric possesses knowledge that transcends the master's understanding of them. The true desire of the hysteric is to secretly seek to dominate the master instead. In light of this Lacanian reinterpretation of Marx's proletariat, it is important to recognize that the proletariat can evolve into a hysterical proletariat. This concept addresses the enigmatic signifier that surpasses the master's comprehension of it. The hysterical proletariat will manifest as the specter of the proletariat that ultimately returns to haunt Marx.

Marx's vision of communism overlooks the psychoanalytic aspects of hysterical existence. In its current form, Marx's communist ideal fails to recognize how the leader of a communist society does not truly govern the proletariat.

This oversight is a symptom of Marx's thinking, of which he remains unaware. Psychoanalysis addresses this issue to enhance the understanding of Marxism and urges it to develop its existing theories. The hysterical existence of the proletariat reveals that they often desire a master in a communist society. However, this master lacks a deep understanding of the proletariat. Consequently, there exists a knowledge gap; while the proletariat may possess profound insights, the master cannot effectively govern until the communist world becomes a terrain of impossible politics. In terms of the proletariat's hysterical existence within a communist framework, psychoanalytic caution suggests that Marxism should not be overly confident in the collective role of the proletariat, as this might not contribute to the stabilization of a communist society. Therefore, what threatens Marx's vision of communism is not merely the emergence of a new master who imposes a repressive regime. Instead, it is the hysterical existence of the proletariat that yearns for a new master – one who ultimately becomes an ineffective sovereign. This situation arises because the proletariat takes pleasure in recognizing the master's ignorance of their true nature.

In terms of similarities between Lacan and Marx, Lacan's hysterical existence can be likened to Marx's proletariat. The proletariat embodies hysterical existence as its desire is not to be governed by the capitalist. However, there are significant divergences; this hysterical proletariat transcends the proletariat imaginary presented by Marx. The envisioned communist reality described by Marx may collapse due to this hysterical proletariat. There are two primary reasons supporting this notion. First, the hysterical proletariat manifests as a failure of the master to maintain control, which ultimately leads to a significant error within the communist universe. Second, this error does not stem solely from the repressive regimes of figures like Lenin, Mao, Stalin, and other revisionists. Because of Marx's lack of psychoanalytic insight, it can be argued that Marx inadvertently creates a symptom in his conceptualization of the proletariat. His initial focus centers on the class conflict, characterizing the struggle between the proletariat and bourgeoisie. Marx tends to position the bourgeoisie as the singular symptom of capitalism, while the proletariat, though diverse, is regarded as the main agent for the establishment of the communist universe. His analysis of capitalism simplifies the struggle into a structural division between the proletariat and the bourgeoisie, effectively propelling the proletariat to become a specter of communism meant to haunt the bourgeoisie. Marx states:

> It is high time that Communists should openly, In the face of the whole world, publish their views, their aims, their tendencies, and meet this nursery tale of the Specter of Communism with a Manifesto of the party itself. To this end, Communists of various nationalities have assembled in London, and sketched the following Manifesto, to be published in the English, French, German, Italian, Flemish, and Danish languages.
>
> (Marx and Engels, 2004, p. 19)

It is evident from the passage that Marx lacks psychoanalytic awareness regarding the existence of a hysterical proletariat within the communist framework. This hysterical condition of the proletariat conflicts with Marx's optimistic vision of communism. This representation of the hysterical existence of the proletariat takes on a mystical quality for the ruling class, serving as a symptom of Marx's broader communist ideology. This notion introduces a latent symptom that parallels Marx's explicit critique of the symptoms of capitalism. Marx primarily focuses on the structural antagonism between the proletariat and the bourgeoisie. He argues that the bourgeoisie, in alliance with religious authority, employs violence to suppress the specter of communism. As he states, "All the Powers of old Europe have entered into a holy alliance to exorcize the specter: Pope and Czar, Metternich and Guizot, French radicals and German police-spies" (Marx and Engels, 2004, p. 19). At the same time, Marx urges the proletariat to awaken from the history of elitist capitalist domination, culminating in the formation of class consciousness among the working class. At this point, it is important to note that the relationship between history and class consciousness plays a significant role in the theoretical perspective of traditional Marxism.

In contrast, if the proletariat embodies hysterical existence, this raises critical awareness regarding Marx and traditional Marxism in relation to history and class consciousness. Marx and Engels famously asserted that "the history of all hitherto existing society is the history of class struggles" (Marx and Engels, 2004, p. 21). The class consciousness of the proletariat is vital and indispensable for the politics of emancipation. However, this theoretical framework of Marxism overlooks a psychoanalytic perspective, which suggests that the proletariat may still develop hysterical tendencies even within a communist society. This psychoanalytic viewpoint offers a cautionary note for Marxism. In a communist world, society will continue to reflect a history of struggles. A new communist leader may not be repressive but rather one who fails to govern effectively due to the proletariat's tendency to obscure the truth from the ruling authority. In a capitalist context, the history and class consciousness serve as a specter that haunts capitalists. Conversely, in a communist setting, it is the hysterical proletariat that becomes a specter haunting the communist regime. This specter represents the uncanny presence that challenges both Marx and traditional Marxism.

A hysterical subject: the demand for mastery and the haunting of Marx

Demanding herself a master

The subject denotes a negation arising from the ego. The ego is shaped by what Lacan calls the "desire of the Other". In this context, the Other implies the desire embedded within capitalism itself. In this internal division of the subject, a distinction arises between the confused self, identified as the ego, and a speculative truth of the self, referred to as the *Cogito*. Understanding this ontology of subjectivity as a form of internal splitting is crucial for re-examining Marx's concept of the proletariat.

The phrase "demanding herself a master" captures the essence of the term "hysteric" as the subject. This was evident on June 10, 1970. After being freed from the extreme interference of the left-wing students, Lacan provided an excellent explanation of the diagram of the hysteric discourse (see Figure 3.1). According to Lacan's description, the barred subject ($) represents the position of agency, and this corresponds to a location of desire. Below the barred subject is the place of truth, which is occupied by the *objet a*. This signifies that the truth concerning the barred subject is articulated through an algebraic framework, with the *objet a* referring to the non-relationship inherent in every discourse. This concept is particularly significant because, in the hysteric discourse, the *objet a* represents the location of truth that is associated with surplus, particularly the surplus-enjoyment. It is the *objet a* that makes the hysteric deviate from the master discourse, which illustrates the master's mapping of knowledge and the identification of truth. In other words, the *objet a* within the hysteric discourse emerges as an uncharted territory, distinctly separate from the mapped cognition associated with the master discourse.

To explore the diagram further, once the barred subject takes over the position of agency from the master, the barred subject becomes the hysteric. This clearly represents the hysteric as a subject resisting the knowledge of the master. Most importantly, at the point of truth, this agency can even push the master (S_1) to the edge of the other, located in the top right-hand corner of the diagram. The

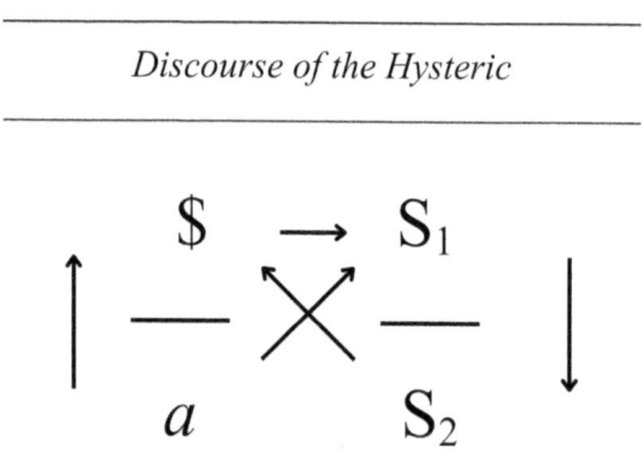

Figure 3.1 Discourse of the hysteric.

Source: Figure adapted from Daniela, D., and Carlos Gomez Camarena. (2022). 'Annex II. What is *matheme*? Four Discourses and Mathematics in Lacan', in *The Marx Through Lacan Vocabulary: A Compass for Libidinal and Political Economies*. Edited by Christina Soto Van Der Plas et al. London and New York: Routledge. p. 289.

master's production of knowledge (S_2) no longer occupies the space of truth because the *objet a* – serving as non-relationship to the master discourse and this is the speculative truth of the hysteric – replaces it. The master's knowledge is intertwined with the Other's question that the subject is compelled to answer. This question is not only ambiguous; it prompts the subject to seek their own desire and locate the *objet a,* which seeks the possible truth of that desire.

The question posed to the subject is "*Che vuoi?*" or "What do you want?" (Lacan, 2006b, p. 690). This question requires careful interpretation. Based on Lacan's original insight, it arises from the perspective of the Other, rather than being a self-directed inquiry by the subject. This question is linked to the concept of the mirror stage. In the stage of early Lacan, the mirror stage represents the relationship between the desire of the Other, the subject, and the potential fragmentation of the subject's own desire, especially in relation to the hysteric. With the question "What do you want?", the Other assesses whether the subject's desire – shaped by the Other since the mirror stage – remains cohesive. However, the subject as the hysteric, in search of "the path of his own desire", does not answer this question based on material satisfaction, which could include objects, relationships, lust, love, or other desires imposed by the Other. Yearning for these tangible things imposed by the Other does not constitute a proper response to "*Che vuoi?*" Since the stage of early Lacan, the question is inverted with the help of the analyst. Thus, "What do you want?" transforms into "What does he want from me?" (Lacan, 2006b, p. 690) or "What does the Other want from me?" Importantly, the subject as the hysteric responds to this inquiry without yielding to the desire of the Other but rather expresses a resistance to this demand.

The discourse of the hysteric is often viewed as somewhat revolutionary – demanding herself a master – because the authority of the master figure is diminished and marginalized. As a result, the hysteric becomes more active and can even assume the role of the master themselves. It is important to critically reflect on the idea that the hysteric silently demands a new master, which may lead to a repressive one: this notion is uneven when considering Lacan's broad explanation of hysteric discourse:

> Let's now take the hysteric's discourse as it is articulated – place the $ on the top left-hand corner, the S_1 on the right, the S_2 underneath, the small *a* in the place of truth. It cannot be the case, either, that the hysteric's division, symptomatic tearing apart, is motivated as the production of knowledge [savoir]. Her truth is that she has to be the objet *a* in order to be desired. The objet *a* is a bit thin, at the end of the day, although, of course, men go crazy about it and they are unable even to suspect that they could get by with anything else – another sign of the impotence that covers the most subtle of all impossibilities.
>
> (Lacan, 2007f, pp. 175–176)

According to the diagram noted by Lacan, the truth of the hysteric serves as the catalyst for desire when viewed from the perspective of the master. This truth is represented as a missing signifier, something that is deemed necessary to be desired but which is ontologically absent from the master's knowledge (S_2). Lacan's formulation suggests that the hysteric's motivation to disrupt the master's authority (S_1) stems from a divergence from the knowledge imparted to her by the master. The hysteric is typically portrayed as a woman, while men or the master becomes obsessed with it. However, the master is unable to attain the hysteric's truth. This situation represents a sign of the impotence that conceals the most subtle of all impossibilities, which pertains not to the hysteric but to the master. Thus, the hysteric's desire, when seen from the master's perspective, represents an impossibility for the master; however, this interpretation is insufficient. It is actually the subject as the hysteric who occupies the master position.

The hysteric's desire represents an impossibility within the master discourse; this interpretation tends to be repetitive and lacks critical examination. To enhance the interpretative depth, it is important to consider that once a hysteric assumes the master position and gains control of a master-signifier, she achieves a status of lordship, shedding her previous role of subjugation (Lacan, 2007e, p. 94). However, a significant concern regarding hysterics emerges from their new role as masters. Driven by a desire rooted in non-satisfaction rather than impossibility, when a hysteric becomes a master and exerts control over statecraft, she personifies a figure that continually dissatisfies and displeases – whether regarding things, people, the existing regime, or even herself. This creates a psychological contradiction, as her dissatisfaction is closely tied to her own desires.

From the perspective of the hysteric, there are two important points to consider. The first is that the hysteric is aware of her desires and of what she lacks; this awareness is not beyond her reach. The second point follows from the first: the hysteric experiences dissatisfaction with her desires. This dissatisfaction creates another significant problem. While the hysteric's desires are attainable for her, she simultaneously feels unsatisfied with them. In short, it is essential to distinguish between *not knowing what one desires* and *knowing what one desires but feeling dissatisfied with it*. To clarify, not knowing what one desires leads to the Other imposing desires onto the subject. In contrast, when a person knows what they truly desire – knowing what one desires – it opens up another dimension of desire for the subject. This allows their desires to diverge from those imposed by the Other. However, the subject realizes and feels that achieving these desires is still far from being fulfilled. This is not viewed as an impossibility, as seen in the discourse of the master; instead, it represents the discourse of the hysteric.

In other words, the most paradoxical issue involves those who assert that the hysteric's desire is impossible. While this perspective seems valid at first glance, it does not truly reflect the hysteric's position. Instead, it reflects a limited understanding of the master in relation to the hysteric. Therefore, the claim that the hysteric's desire is undefinable and impossible is contentious and open to debate. Drawing on Lacan's original insights, the hysteric possesses "her truth" (Lacan, 2007f, p. 175). This implies that the subject as the hysteric may begin her journey with a sense of lacking truth but can ultimately overcome this struggle by seeking and understanding the truth of her desire – if successful. If hysteric transitions from a sense of lack to the possibility of knowing her own truth, it involves discovering and identifying the unconscious desires within herself. This does not mean that the hysteric's desire is impossible; rather, it indicates that she experiences ongoing dissatisfaction with her desires, even though she holds a master position. Consequently, this dissatisfaction leads her truth and desire to become the *objet a*, even to herself, which represents a non-relationship to herself; but this dynamic ultimately makes her more desirable to men.

Proletariat: the hysterical subject as the master that haunts Marx

Rather than viewing an optimistic and harmonious relationship between Lacan and Marx, re-examining Marx's work through a psychoanalytic lens reveals an alternative perspective. The proletariat can be seen as the hysterical subject who demands to occupy a position of mastery. This idea of the proletariat as a hysterical subject is an alternative to the definition of the proletariat under capitalism, which views them as laborers who exchange their labor force and time for disproportionately low wages. This notion also has the potential to disrupt Marx's vision of a communist society from within. Although the proletariat is an agent of revolution, what poses a threat to the communist ideal imagined by Marx is the possibility of the proletariat, as the hysterical subject, ascending to a position of mastery that could dismantle the entire structure. This hysterical proletariat would likely remain dissatisfied even in a classless society, serving as a cautionary note to Marx and traditional Marxism. It suggests that historical contingencies will persist, even within Marx's concept of a classless society.

To understand the issue discussed earlier, it is important to examine this quote from Marx and Engels:

> In what relation do the Communists stand to the proletariats as a whole? The Communists do not form a separate party opposed to the other working-class parties. They have no interests separate and apart from those of proletariat as a whole. They do not set up any sectarian principles of their own, by which to shape and mould the proletariat movement.
>
> (Marx and Engels, 2004, p. 37)

In a reinterpretation of Marx's concept of communism through a Lacanian lens, the argument can be made that the proletariat, often described as hysterical subject, embodies the true essence of communism. This interpretation highlights the connection between Marx's and Lacan's theories, viewing the proletariat as a hysterical subject in search of mastery. The term "communist" refers to the proletariat, particularly the working-class parties that lead communism. However, this shared perspective between Marx and Lacan has its limitations, as it tends to overlook the limitations in Marx's understanding of the proletariat. When considering the proletariat's subject as a hysterical proletariat, it becomes clear that they understand what is desirable for them. This desire is not impossible, but over time, they may find it no longer satisfying. Given this understanding of the hysteric, how does Marx ensure that the proletariat, as he envisions it, will not be separated from his vision of communism?

If the proletariat as a hysterical subject is gendered as female, then their contingent desires may become something that Marx, as a man, would "go crazy about it" (Lacan, 2007f, pp. 175–176). Marx, who speaks from the position of the master, will ultimately show "signs of impotence that cover the most subtle of all impossibilities" (Lacan, 2007f, pp. 175–176). This is due to the possibility that the hysterical proletariat may later oppose a classless society, influenced by their differing interpretations of communism, which contrast with Marx's original vision. Therefore, it is not communism that creates a world of egalitarianism but rather egalitarian worlds within the singularity of communism that fulfill themselves through a positive negation of Marx's monolithic vision. In a Lacanian interpretation of Marx, the issues discussed represent Marx's *objet a*, which refers to the non-relationship that Marx fails to acknowledge in his initial discourse about the proletariat. This is particularly significant when considering how this hysterical proletariat eventually attains a position of authority or master status. Metaphorically, there is a gender gap between the vision of a communist world held by the hysterical proletariat – a vision that is mystical and resonates deeply with feminine desires – and Marx's interpretation, which is rooted in male dominance. While Marx may initially be surprised by the proletariat's temporary admiration for him, there is a risk that, over time, Marx will come to see the hysterical proletariat as a precious treasure, the most desirable object, which is sought "in order to be desired" by a male. This perception arises from Marx's limited understanding of her, the hysterical proletariat. Slavoj Žižek characterizes that the hysteric "believes in the hidden existence of a totalizing knowledge about the truth of her *objet a*, although she has never had the least experience of it" (Žižek, 1994, p. 131). Following Žižek's perspective, it can be said that the hysterical proletariat assumes that there is an inherent truth about themselves – specifically regarding communism, which differs from Marx's conception – that can be represented in Lacanian terms as the *objet a* internalized within themselves. However, this belief is paradoxical because they have never had any direct, phenomenological experiences related to this sense of truth.

In the position of the master, there exists a will to power and a need to dominate, which can lead to a proletariat as a hysterical subject that finds the previously satisfactory communist world no longer adequate. By dissociating from it, they inadvertently face a significant challenge: they may not have a clear vision of what a desired communist world actually looks like. While some may have faith in the existence of alternative communist worlds beyond Marx's original vision, the primary issue is that they have never experienced such worlds. The absence of experience presents a challenge within the communist framework and highlights what Marx may have unconsciously overlooked – his *objet a* – and the symptoms he neglects in his analysis of the proletariat and the specter of communism. Although situated in a position of mastery, the hysteric's desire is notably contingent and appears unfulfilled. As Lacan points out, it symbolizes a state of non-satisfaction: "it is the basis on which we can understand how the hysteric symbolizes the initial non-satisfaction" (Lacan, 2007g, p. 74). The uncanny presence that haunts Marx's vision of a communist world, in relation to his idea of the proletariat, arises from this hysterical proletariat. The fundamental challenge lies in the fact that "the impossibility of satisfying desire is reflexively inverted into the desire for non-satisfaction, the desire to maintain itself unsatisfied" (Žižek, 2000, p. 345).

In Lacanian terms, a philosophical and psychoanalytic issue arises from the distinction between the ego and the subject. This distinction challenges the dialectic between the ego, which represents the individual as a reflection of the desire of the Other, and the emergence of self-fragmentation that breaks away from that desire, where the "I" or *Cogito* expresses thoughts from a perspective where speculative truth is explored. This dialectic is based on the division between the ego – characterized as a neurotic reproduction of alienation – and a hysterical denial of such hallucinatory false image. As a result, the Lacanian subject is perceived as an existential being that is fundamentally out-of-joint. One can position the hysterical proletariat not within the realm of the desire of the Other but on the side of the subject. If one considers Marx's vision of a communist society as a reflective of the desire of the Other, then the hysterical proletariat, in achieving self-autonomy, is prompted by the psychoanalytic question known as *Che Voui?* or What does the Other want from me? Therefore, it is inadequate to merely define Marx as a male hysteric, implying that his political ideology is the true adversary of capitalism. Instead, the hysterical proletariat raises critical questions that create an epistemological gap between themselves and the ideas of Marx and Engels. For example, in their manifesto, the hysterical proletariat, as a subject, might ask, "What do Karl Marx and Friedrich Engels want from me?"

The concept of proletariat as a hysterical subject can be integrally related to the ideological call for "working men of all countries, unite!" (Marx and Engels, 2004, p. 64). However, once this proletariat rises to power, it may transform into a haunting specter that Marx did not anticipate. This grotesque entity signifies a departure from Marx and Engels' vision of a communist utopia, and it is not limited to Leninist regimes or similar systems. While Marx identified the specter of communism haunting Europe, the hysterical proletariat becomes the specter that haunts Marx and his vision of a communist world. This represents Marx's unconscious. This unconscious is ever-present, functioning like the figures of the King and Queen in Velázquez's *Las Meninas*, who seem to stand just outside the pictorial frame. Although their appearances are subtly underrepresented and ambiguous, their essence is always implied and intended by the painter from the very beginning. Similarly, as a subject, the hysterical proletariat is continuously present – though shadowed and virtually absent – in Marx's writings on the proletariat and his vision of a communist society, but Marx is unaware of it. Understanding this unconscious aspect requires thoughtful interpretation. By revisiting Marx's texts through the lens of Lacan's psychoanalytic concepts, one can uncover valuable insights, revealing Marx's unconscious and the symptoms related to it.

A sublime hysteric: the surplus-crisis, politics, and the proletariat

Surplus-crisis

It is emphasized in the main thesis of proletariat discourse that the emancipatory politics of the proletariat is grounded in anti-capitalism. Unlike in Marx's time, the ongoing crises of global capitalism are no longer one-dimensional. They represent a surplus-crisis. This crisis is inevitably multifaceted, arising from the negative consequences generated by global labor relations, gender dynamics, racial issues, and ecological challenges that universally affect us all (Bieler, 2025). Considering these multiple crises in relation to the reproduction of capitalism reveals that the issues extend beyond the traditional sphere of proletariat and capitalist relationships. They also encompass social dimensions such as gender, race, and ecological crises.

Thus, a new philosophy that articulates a principle of struggle is urgently needed. In the context of the surplus crisis, there is a movement to redefine class struggle and the labor movement. Andreas Bieler argues that forging a broad alliance with trade unions, feminist groups, environmental organizations, developmental organizations, social movements, and citizens' committees is crucial in the fight against capitalist exploitation (Bieler, 2025, pp. 915–932). He emphasizes that "it is through these moments of class struggle that shared understandings of social justice may emerge, even if people come from different backgrounds" (Bieler, 2025, pp. 915–932). Bieler's argument, which focuses on various forms of resistance to capitalism, is both timely and refreshing. He avoids glorifying the idea of multiple sites of plural struggles, often advocated by the Lacanian Left and Left populism, as an ultimate emancipatory goal.

Bieler's perspective stands in stark contrast to the politics of Lacanian Left and Left populism, which have played a role in the emergence of cultural wokeism in contemporary society. Influenced by Ernesto Laclau's ideas, Left populism includes a group of thinkers who focus on themes of abundance but feel a lack of social belonging. While they critique capitalism, they have yet to unify into forming a coherent global movement to challenge it. Instead, they support "alternative life-forms" through a strategy of pluralization, which values the virtues of agonism and critical responsiveness (Tønder and Thomassen, 2005, p. 7). Their intense focus on the politics of difference can sometimes lead to societal fragmentation and may overlook the importance of a psychoanalytic critique of capitalism. Additionally, it is important to consider what Žižek describes as "the extreme case of *jouissance*" (Žižek, 2023 p. 192), or the excessive enjoyment associated with global capitalism. In this context, surplus-enjoyment refers to a type of pleasure that is intertwined with pain – a pleasurable experience that often requires a painful sacrifice to gain and maintain that pleasure. Surplus-enjoyment is not solely connected to the subject's death drive. A critical aspect of surplus-enjoyment, as emphasized by the late Lacan, is the idea of experiencing pain within pleasure (Lacan, 2007d, p. 46). For example, capitalism cannot achieve an excessive level of enjoyment without causing significant negative consequences or severe pain on a global scale. The subject realizes that pleasure becomes a lack. They repeat the same action until the pleasure becomes surplus, but the excess of pleasure cannot avoid the severe pain and loss it generates to themselves and others.

Similarly, Žižek's article distinctly separates itself from both the Lacanian Left or Left populism. He argues that their focus is insufficiently directed toward the universality of global capitalism and its associated crises. Without attaining true emancipation, they are overly concerned with a Laclauian approach that emphasizes the competitive struggle for discursive hegemony, in which Žižek criticizes as "a discourse-analysis that focuses on the competitive game for discursive hegemony" (Žižek, 2023, p. 191). Žižek states that

> the extreme case of *jouissance today* is, of course, the prospect of apocalypse in all its versions (pandemic, ecological catastrophes, nuclear war, dissolution of social order), including total knowledge itself: wouldn't it be apocalyptic to gain direct access to another's stream of thoughts?
>
> (Žižek, 2023, p. 192)

Without considering apocalyptic phenomena or the crisis of surplus in global capitalism, a political approach that limits itself to merely articulating discourse in favor of multiple opposing political agendas will ultimately undermine its own potential for emancipation.

A sublime hysteric: the essence and its politics

The term "politics" emphasizes liberation from capitalism and its surplus crisis. This aligns with Lacan's call to "exit capitalist discourse", which resonates with Marx's vision of the proletariat as a revolutionary force in the pursuit of emancipation. To understand the characteristics of the proletariat in relation to Lacan's concept of the hysteric, it is essential to link the proletariat with Lacan's sublime hysteric.

What is the essence of the sublime hysteric? The sublime hysteric refers to a desire that arises in the discourse of the hysteric after rejecting the contributions of the other two repressive discourses – master discourse and university discourse. This rejection prompts the hysteric to "designate for us as being that of truth" (Lacan, 2007h, p. 35). As a philosophical-psychoanalyst, Lacan positions himself within the analyst discourse. As the analyst, Lacan observes that the hysteric actively negates the dominance of the master discourse's production of knowledge, as well as the university discourse that supports the educational system propagating this dominant knowledge of the master. In contrast to these two discourses, the hysteric emerges as critical of them, seeking her own form of speculative truth.

On December 17, 1969, Lacan characterized Hegel as the example of "the most sublime of hysterics" (Lacan, 2007h, p. 35). Indeed, the essence of sublime hysteric converges with Hegel's explanation in *The Phenomenology of Spirit*. The self is the "sense-certainty", which "appears to be the truest knowledge" (Hegel, 1977, p. 58). The sense-certainty is related to a negation from the immediate ground of being; it seeks opposition to something given as essential, notably, the background of its existence. As Hegel (1977, p. 62) states, the true meaning of "I" does not refer to the continuity in the background of the given essential. Phenomenology emphasizes something beyond the discourses that reveal the appearances of truth. By negating a foundation of self-certainty to embrace sense-certainty, the meaning of hysteric aims to attain knowledge within herself. Consequently, the knowledge that has traditionally been invested in the master is dissected and ultimately dismantled. In this sense, the sublime hysteric must endure resistance and seek emancipation, not only from a political regime but also from the knowledge constructed by the master. This struggle culminates in a dialectic against the master discourse, allowing her to achieve a sense of enjoyment beyond a deterministic ground of being, and resonates with Hegel's sense-certainty (Lacan, 2007h, p. 35).

The proletariat as a sublime hysteric

In the context of the surplus-crisis of global capitalism, the proletariat can be seen as a sublime hysteric. While Marx often views the proletariat as a driving force for political revolution, he neglects to consider it from a psychoanalytic perspective. This viewpoint reflects a limitation in Marx's analysis. It invites a comparison between Lacan and Marx, illustrating both their connections and differences, and suggesting a potential for Lacan's ideas to extend beyond those of Marx: Lacan beyond Marx. From an empirical standpoint, Bieler's call for a divergence of social actors to unite in a new class struggle embodies a significant expression of this collective nature of the sublime hysterical proletariat.

However, when delving into theoretical discussions, two key characteristics emerge regarding the proletariat as a psychoanalytically defined sublime hysteric. First, the proletariat, as a sublime hysteric, can reclaim the status of speculative truth by rejecting the dominant master discourse. Second, in contrast to university discourse, the proletariat functions as a sublime hysteric that distances itself from what Lacan refers to as "I-cracy" (Lacan, 2007i, p. 63).

In the first characteristic, the proletariat is seen as a sublime hysteric in relation to the master's discourse. It embodies knowledge that goes beyond the confines of this discourse. This is why Lacan refers to the proletariat, without hesitation, as *objet a* – the non-relationship that is fundamental within the master's discourse. Although the proletariat is compelled to perceive themselves merely as victims of exploitation, this overwhelming influence of the master's discourse tends to undermine their status as holders of speculative truth. As Lacan explains:

> The proletariat is not simply exploited, he has been stripped off his function of knowledge. The so-called liberation of the slave has had, as always, other corollaries. It's not merely progressive. It is progressive only at the price of a deprivation. . . . The renewed emphasis on the knowledge of the exploited seems to me to be very profoundly motivated structurally.
>
> (Lacan, 2007c, p. 149)

In the passage, Lacan aims to identify the proletariat by dismantling the notion of exploitation that is dominated by the master – essentially, the slave deprived of their status as a bearer of truth in the master's discourse. Lacan perceives the proletariat as a hysterical being whose potential for truth is redeemable. Gaining knowledge about the proletariat as a sublime hysteric is a progressive step, albeit at the cost of their almost total deprivation. This emphasizes the status of the proletariat as a sublime hysteric. The knowledge derived from this position – one that is not identical to the experience of exploitation – is something that should be encouraged.

In the second characteristic, university discourse reveals a connection between the master's production of knowledge and its dissemination throughout society. The sublime hysteric serves as the *objet a* that is inherent in university discourse. Lacan refers to this situation using his own concept of *lalangue*, a self-invention of words that operates independently of conventional meaning, calling it "I-cracy" (Lacan, 2007i, p. 63). The term "I-cracy" signifies "the I as it is transcendental, but, equally, insofar as it is illusory" (Lacan, 2007i, p. 62). This context requires the sublime hysteric to break free from the illusion of I-cracy, particularly as it relates to university discourse. I-cracy functions as a non-totalized signifier, representing something that remains obscured within university discourse. This alludes to the unthought, or the aspect of "what the university discourse is unable to eliminate from the place in which its truth is found" (Lacan, 2007i, p. 63). The objective of identifying with the *objet a* inherent in

I-cracy is to save truth (Lacan, 2007i, p. 63). At this stage, it is clear that Lacan is not against philosophy, contrary to common misconceptions. He states, "I am attacking philosophy? That's greatly exaggerated" (Lacan, 2007c, p. 146).

Lacan's concept of capitalist discourse addresses the capitalist subject and the consumerist subject, highlighting the sense of unfulfillment that leads to surplus-enjoyment, as discussed in Chapter 1. This capitalist discourse is often repeated within Lacanian-Marxist communities, but it tends to overlook the fact that Lacan also connects capitalism to the university discourse, which he refers to as the realm of I-cracy. He states, "Let's now ask how this society called capitalist society can afford to allow itself a relaxation of the university discourse" (Lacan, 2007f, p. 168). How can one uncover the truth behind this university discourse? Lacan suggests that the university discourse is flawed: it has an inherent deficiency. To preserve the truth, one must address "a reform in its hole" (Lacan, 2007f, p. 168), ultimately leading to the dethronement of the I-cracy sustained by the university discourse. What exactly does Lacan mean by this "hole" that requires reform? He explains that "at the level of the university discourse, the *objet a* comes to occupy a position that is in play each time it moves, the place more or less tolerable exploitation" (Lacan, 2007f, p. 178). In this context, the *objet a* symbolizes all those who endure a tolerable form of exploitation. The sublime hysteric carries the responsibility of reforming this hole by challenging the acceptance of tolerable exploitation. The goal of the proletariat, viewed through the lens of the sublime hysteric, is to uncover the truth of their experience, liberated from the illusions propagated by the university discourse.

This conceptualization of the proletariat as a sublime hysteric disrupts the established norms of university discourse, creating an uneasy relationship with the views of Marx and Engels. They argue that in a communist society, the education system will be freed from capitalist influence. According to them, the goal of communism is to "rescue education from the influence of the ruling class" (Marx and Engels, 2004, p. 44). They assert that the proletariat must utilize the knowledge and tools provided by the capitalists to challenge the capitalist system. Marx and Engels further claim that the bourgeoisie itself supplies the proletariat with the means of political and general education, essentially equipping the proletariat with "weapons for fighting the bourgeoisie" (Marx and Engels, 1848, 2004, p. 33). However, this assertion raises a critical question: what is the speculative inner truth of the proletariat? Marx and Engels seem to overlook this inquiry, which sets them apart from Lacan's portrayal of the proletariat as a sublime hysteric within university discourse. In essence, it is ambiguous whether Marx and Engels genuinely seek to uncover the truth of the proletariat or merely view them as instrumental in a teleological revolution, without any sincere reflection on their deeper truth.

Marx and Engels seem to prefer understanding the proletariat solely through their own ideological frameworks and concepts, which undermines the true nature of the proletariat – a truth that remains elusive to them. This perspective contrasts with Lacan's view of the proletariat as a sublime hysteric, whose mission is to save the truth about the proletariat. In the context of university discourse, where there is a general consensus on tolerable exploitation, Lacan argues that capitalism thrives within the university system. This success is attributed to the I-cracy prevalent in university discourse, where everyone appears to accept a repressive regime until the situation becomes untenable and necessary reforms seem impossible. Lacan explicitly addresses the students, stating, "You are all an *objet a*, insofar as you are lined up there" (Lacan, 2007f, p. 178). He continues to elaborate on this idea:

> You are the product of the university, and you prove that you are the surplus-value, even if only in this respect – which you not only consent to, but which you also applaud – and I see no reason to object – which is that you leave here, yourselves equivalent to more or fewer credit points. You come here to gain credit points for yourselves. You leave here stamped, "credit points."
>
> (Lacan, 2007a, p. 201)

In Lacan's statement, students attend university primarily to earn "credit points", becoming stamped with qualifications. Upon graduation, many leave without truly understanding their true identities. As they transition into what may be the future proletariat, they are suddenly faced with the challenge of becoming the sublime hysteric – questioning the university discourse, who am I for you? This question stems from a desire to uncover their own speculative truths. However, the university discourse, aligned with capitalism, does not encourage them to ask this crucial question. Instead, students become products of the university system. While the institution generates surplus-value from students' tuition fees, those students focus solely on accumulating credit points, rarely engaging in critical self-reflection about their identities desired by the Other – the university discourse – which Lacan critiques as an instance of I-cracy.

Lacan may be unaware that his reflections are closely linked to the concept of the "neoliberal university". Igea Troiani and Claudia Dutson (2021) critique the neoliberal university as an illusory space. The I-cracy of the neoliberal university promises to "increase performance – measurable in ultimately economic terms, imposing a new auditable disciplining, and quickening pace, of learning, thinking, and working" (Troiani and Dutson, 2021). However, this illusion is closely tied to capitalism. The operations of the neoliberal university are not separate from capitalist logic, as they are "encouraged to develop links with industry and business in a series of new venture partnerships" (Olssen and Peters, 2005). Troiani and Dutson also argue for a need to resist, rethink, and reclaim the space for learning, thinking, and working. This political message aims to save the university from the prevailing neoliberal ideology. It also intersects with the struggles of the proletariat, who act as a sublime hysteric and must work to reform the flawed university system. This represents an initial step or a starting point toward seeking their own speculative truth.

In conclusion, this chapter explores the concept of the hysterical proletariat by revisiting Marx's idea of the specter of communism through a Lacanian psychoanalytic lens. The hysterical proletariat emerges from a hysterical psyche, which is described as aphasic. This state of hysterical existence reflects a failure of the ruling class to maintain control, resulting in ontological inconsistency within Marx's communist imaginary. As a result, the proletariat, regarded as a hysterical subject, may find it difficult to envision a new communist world. They may believe that this world could differ from Marx's vision, yet they lack concrete experiences of alternative realities. Politically, this connects to the proletariat's desire to reform the flawed university system that is dominated by capitalism, which serves as a crucial starting point in their quest for speculative truth.

Reference list

Bieler, A. (2025). 'Confronting Multiple Global Crises: A Political Economy Approach for the Twenty-first Century', *Globalizations*, 22(6), 915–932.

Fierens, C. (2022). '"I Think" in the Psychoanalytic Discourse or Cogito and the Psychoanalytic Discourse', in *Lacan and Other Heresies: Lacanian Psychoanalytic Writings*. Edited by Linda Clifton. New York and Oxon: Routledge.

Freud, S., and Joseph Breuer. (2004). *Studies in Hysteria*. Translated by Nicola Luckhurst. London: Penguin Books.

Hegel, G. (1977). 'Consciousness', in *Phenomenology of Spirit*. Translated by A.V. Miller. Oxford: Oxford University Press.

Hegel, G. (2010a). 'Appearance', in *The Science of Logic*. Translated by George Di Giovanni. Cambridge: Cambridge University Press.

Hegel, G. (2010b). 'Quantity', in *The Science of Logic*. Translated by George Di Giovanni. Cambridge: Cambridge University Press.

Lacan, J. (1986a). 'Of the Network of Signifiers', in *The Seminar of Jacques Lacan Book XI: The Four Fundamental Concepts of Psychoanalysis*. Edited by Jacques-Alain Miller. Translated by Alan Sheridan. London: Penguin Books.

Lacan, J. (1986b). 'The Eye and the Gaze', in *The Seminar of Jacques Lacan Book XI: The Four Fundamental Concepts of Psychoanalysis*. Edited by Jacques-Alain Miller. Translated by Alan Sheridan. London: Penguin Books.

Lacan, J. (1991). 'Introduction to the Commentaries on Freud's Papers on Technique', in *The Seminar of Jacques Lacan Book I: Freud's Papers on Technique*. Edited by Jacques-Alain Miller. Translated by John Forrester. London and New York: W.W. Norton & Company.

Lacan, J. (2006a). 'Seminar on "The Purloined Letter", in *Écrits: The First Complete Edition in English*. Translated by Bruce Fink. London and New York: W.W. Norton & Company.

Lacan, J. (2006b). 'The Subversion of the Subject and the Dialectic of Desire in the Freudian Unconscious', in *Écrits: The First Complete Edition in English*. Translated by Bruce Fink. London and New York: W.W. Norton & Company.

Lacan, J. (2007a). 'Analyticon', in *The Seminar of Jacques Lacan Book XVII: The Other Side of Psychoanalysis*. Translated by Russell Grigg. London and New York: W.W. Norton & Company.

Lacan, J. (2007b). 'From myth to structure', in *The Seminar of Jacques Lacan Book XVII: The Other Side of Psychoanalysis*. Translated by Russell Grigg. London and New York: W.W. Norton & Company.

Lacan, J. (2007c). 'Interview on the Steps of the Pantheon', in *The Seminar of Jacques Lacan Book XVII: The Other Side of Psychoanalysis*. Translated by Russell Grigg. London and New York: W.W. Norton & Company.

Lacan, J. (2007d). 'Knowledge, A Means of *Jouissance*', in *The Seminar of Jacques Lacan Book XVII: The Other Side of Psychoanalysis*. Translated by Russell Grigg. London and New York: W.W. Norton & Company.

Lacan, J. (2007e). 'The castrated master', in *The Seminar of Jacques Lacan Book XVII: The Other Side of Psychoanalysis*. Translated by Russell Grigg. London and New York: W.W. Norton & Company.

Lacan, J. (2007f). 'The Impotence of Truth', in *The Seminar of Jacques Lacan Book XVII: The Other Side of Psychoanalysis*. Translated by Russell Grigg. London and New York: W.W. Norton & Company.

Lacan, J. (2007g). 'The Lacanian field', in *The Seminar of Jacques Lacan Book XVII: The Other Side of Psychoanalysis*. Translated by Russell Grigg. London and New York: W.W. Norton & Company.

Lacan, J. (2007h). 'The Master and the Hysteric', in *The Seminar of Jacques Lacan Book XVII: The Other Side of Psychoanalysis*. Translated by Russell Grigg. London and New York: W.W. Norton & Company.

Lacan, J. (2007i). 'Truth, the Sister of *Jouissance*', in *The Seminar of Jacques Lacan Book XVII: The Other Side of Psychoanalysis*. Translated by Russell Grigg. London and New York: W.W. Norton & Company.

Lichtenstein, D. (2018). 'Multiplicity and Rigor in Psychoanalysis', in *Progress in Psychoanalysis: Envisioning the Future of the Profession*. Edited by Steven D. Axelrod, Ronald C. Naso, and Larry M. Rosenberg. New York and Oxon: Routledge.

Marx, K., and Friedrich Engels. (2004). 'Communist Manifesto', in *Karl Marx: Essential Thinkers*. London: CRW Publishing Limited.

Olssen, M., and Peters, M. A. (2005). 'Neoliberalism, Higher Education and the Knowledge Economy: From the Free Market to Knowledge Capitalism', *Journal of Education Policy*, 20(3), 313–345. https://doi.org/10.1080/02680930500108718: Accessed: December 15, 2025.

Tønder, L., and Lasse Thomassen. (2005). *Radical Democracy: Politics Between Abundance and Lack*. Manchester and New York: Manchester University Press.

Troiani, I., and Dutson, C. (2021). 'The Neoliberal University as a Space to Learn/Think/Work in Higher Education', *Architecture and Culture*, 9(1), 5–23. https://doi.org/10.1080/20507828.2021.1898836: Accessed: December 15, 2025.

Žižek, S. (1994). *The Metastases of Enjoyment: On Women and Causality*. London and New York: Verso.

Žižek, S. (2000). *The Ticklish Subject: The Absent Centre of Political Ontology*. London and New York: Verso.

Žižek, S. (2014). *The Most Sublime Hysteric: Hegel and Lacan*. Translated by Thomas Scott-Railton. Cambridge and Malden: Polity Press.

Žižek, S. (2023). 'Matrix Resurrections, or Jouissance as a Political Factor', in *Capitalism and the New Political Unconscious: A Philosophy of Immanence*. Translated by Riccardo Panattoni and Fabio Vighi. London and New York: Bloomsbury Academic.

4 Reexamining alienation and commodity fetishism

Proletariat in the vel of alienation and the contradictory principles of the unconscious

This chapter aims to reexamine Karl Marx's concepts of alienation and commodity fetishism, particularly in relation to his understanding of the proletariat. Additionally, the chapter explores Jacques Lacan's idea of the vel of alienation, where he distinguishes between two opposing forms of alienation: the lethal form and the celebrated form. Lacan's vel of alienation presents a dialectical image of alienation that is embedded within the subject of the proletariat. On the one hand, the subject of the proletariat reflects a connection between Marx's notion of alienation – connected to commodity fetishism and the objectification of labor – and Lacan's concept of lethal alienation. On the other, there exists a tension between Marx's understanding of alienation and Lacan's celebrated alienation. Instead of adhering to Marxism's perspective that advocates for overcoming alienation generated by the structural inequalities of capitalism through class consciousness, the subject of the proletariat accepts a celebrated form of alienation.

This chapter is structured around four fundamental dimensions of proletariat discourse: psyche, existence, subject, and politics. The arguments are divided into four main sections. The first section explores alienation based on psychoanalytical concept. It discusses how Lacan develops the idea of alienation, referred to as the vel of alienation, based on his experience of excommunication. The second section focuses on the existence of the proletariat. It examines Marx's analysis of the relationship between the proletariat, commodity fetishism, and alienation. By revisiting Marx's concept of alienation through the lens of Lacan's vel of alienation, it is possible that there is a notable connection between Marx's understanding of alienation and Lacan's notion of lethal alienation. This section also highlights a philosophical dimension that Marx may have overlooked, especially his understanding of philosophy, which is related to changing the world that avoids a mere interpretation of it. Furthermore, the proletariat exhibits a conflict between Marx's alienation and Lacan's more celebrated version, which involves *ex-sistence* and separation.

In the third section, the chapter examines the concepts of the proletariat, subjectivity, and the unconscious. It posits that Lacan's understanding of the

DOI: 10.4324/9781003657781-4

unconscious is not simply confined to repressed thoughts that can be expressed through language. While Marx seems to define proletariat's subjectivity as wage labor, unconscious, which encompasses the contradictory principles, shapes both the proletariat's subjectivity – the subject of the proletariat – and their unconscious in two opposing ways. First, the unconscious compels the proletariat to engage with the desire of the Other, specifically the desires of the capitalist Other. This forces the proletariat to derive pleasure or ego-satisfaction from the existing reality of capitalism. Second, conversely, the unconscious can also function in a contrary manner. It urges the proletariat to become aware of their discontent with capitalism, disassociating them from the desire of the capitalist Other, and encouraging them to see the communist imaginary as an object of desire: the *objet a*, or small o. However, the unconscious operates in a cyclical manner. It can push the proletariat toward anti-capitalist sentiments, yet it can also lead them back to continue working for capitalism. This creates an internal contradiction within both the unconscious and the subjectivity of the proletariat.

In the fourth section, the chapter explores the relationship between the proletariat and politics. Both Lacan and Marx offer critical insights into capitalism, allowing them to diverge from the Lacanian Left or Left populism. Furthermore, the paradoxical nature of the unconscious discussed in the third section, combined with the concept of alienation examined in the first and second sections, can facilitate a constructive dialogue with Marx's and traditional Marxism's views on overcoming alienation involved with fostering class consciousness among the proletariat.

Alienation as a psyche: excommunication and the vel of alienation

Excommunication

In psychology, alienation is understood as a Gestalt concept. It refers to individuals who feel a significant disconnect from the society that influences them. This perspective emphasizes that self-realization is a worthy goal, highlighting both alienated individuals and those who resonate with such social alienation as unfulfilled individuals (Schacht, 1992, p. 4). However, Lacan reinterprets alienation, distancing it from the framework of psychology. Lacan considers alienation to be significant for psychoanalysis and positive for the formation of the subject, stemming from his personal experience of being excommunicated from the International Psychoanalytical Association (IPA) (Lacan, 1986b, p. 3).

Lacan's concept of alienation is closely linked to his experience of excommunication. He suggests that the IPA functions like a religious community, prompting the question: "What is it in that community that is so reminiscent of religious practice?" (Lacan, 1986b, p. 4). Notably, his excommunication became apparent during the first week of Seminar XI, *The Four Fundamental Concepts of*

Psychoanalysis (1964). During this seminar, the audience was informed that his teachings had faced censure from a group known as the Executive Committee of the International Psychoanalytical Association (Lacan, 1986b, p. 3).

The essential aspect of excommunication extends beyond the psychological experience and emotional distress of being expelled from a particular place; it is not merely a repressive emotion. The true nature of excommunication is sublimation. In Lacan's view, he sublimates his mental state of being excommunicated from one oppressive condition to a more liberating one. To a certain extent, his excommunication leads to a new formation of his subjectivity, which embodies the concept of "the lack of the lack that makes the real" (Lacan, 1986e, p. ix). Excommunication, in this sense, represents the Real. The Real is something that tends to "show its antinomy to all verisimilitude" (Lacan, 1986e, p. ix). Consequently, the Real – Lacan's sublimation of excommunication into the Real – becomes something unsignified and mystically unknown to the symbolic authority of the IPA. This examination of excommunication is distinctly different from the concept of alienation, which is defined as a unified Gestalt in social psychology, as discussed earlier.

Lacan's vel of alienation: the lethal form of alienation and the celebrated form of alienation

Lacan's excommunication leads him to introduce the term "vel of alienation" (Lacan, 1986g, p. 211). Following a principle of Hegelian dialectics, Lacan suggests that "the vel of alienation is a matter of choice" (Lacan, 1986g, p. 211). This notion of choice is, in fact, paradoxical. Lacan employs a Hegelian dialectical method to emphasize that "I should indicate here where the Hegelian lure proceeds" (Lacan, 1986h, p. 221). The Hegelian dialectical approach to knowledge acquisition is embedded in Lacan's exploration of alienation. This distinction is crucial as it reveals a divide between lethal alienation, which Lacan associates with "the object of what is called a deal" (Lacan, 1986b, p. 4), and celebrated alienation, linked to Lacan's introduction of "the myth of the lamella" (Lacan, 1986g, p. 205). In essence, while Hegel's dialectic highlights the internal contradictions present within each concept, alienation also embodies an intrinsic contradiction that fuels its essence; the human psyche is no exception to this aspect of Hegel's dialectic. There are two situations that illustrate the vel of alienation as a matter of choice.

In the first choice, the subject chooses to exist meaningfully within the realm of the symbolic order. However, this choice comes at a cost: when the subject makes the decision to belong to the symbolic order, they inevitably risk falling into a domain devoid of meaning. In other words, by aligning themselves with the symbolic order, the subject becomes consumed or devoured by it. This causes alienation, as the subject becomes something that is absent from the symbolic order. As a result, the subject experiences distress and struggles to achieve a true sense of self, feeling as though they are an outsider to their own identity. This condition illustrates the experience of subjects whose lives have fallen outside the official structure of reality. This situation, where the subject's psyche is dominated and demanded for a compliance by the symbolic order, can be referred to as "lethal alienation".

In contrast, there is an alternative choice: the subject can choose to separate from the realm of the symbolic order. Lacan describes what he calls "celebrated alienation" as a liberatory form of alienation (Lacan, 1986g, p. 210). This excommunication leads Lacan to establish an anti-psychoanalytic establishment, positioning himself as a subject of the Real that threatens the symbolic authority of the IPA. In this context, celebrated alienation represents a situation where the subject's psyche seeks to assert itself as the Real, which challenges the symbolic order. The subject forms and revolves around a lack in the symbolic order. The order is ontologically inconsistent, structured by antagonisms, and prevents harmonious relationships (Žižek, 2016, p. 37). Ultimately, it is important to note that Lacan's concept of the vel of alienation, detailed subsequently, is both philosophically and psychoanalytically valuable for rethinking Marx's notion of the proletariat.

The lethal form of alienation

The lethal form of alienation can also be referred to as negative alienation. This concept highlights a "lethal factor" (Lacan, 1986g, p. 213) in which the subject becomes self-destructive. The subject emerges while paradoxically disappearing within the field of the Other. The field of the Other consists of the network of signifiers that produce and shape subjectivity for individuals. Although the Other represents the social realm of language, signifiers, norms, and civilization that are crucial for the constitution of subjectivity, the emergence of subjectivity after this process is both problematic and paradoxical. Currently, lethal alienation highlights the effects of the signifier and its role in shaping specific worldviews, particularly through information, communication, and social network platforms. This often leads to the dehumanization of the subject, reducing the subject "to being no more than a signifier" and "to petrify the subject in the same movement in which it calls the subject to function, to speak, as subject" (Lacan, 1986g, p. 207). The subject as a signifier of speaking being is at risk to be "a lure in or even as an obstruction to the revelation of truth, it is insofar as it serves as a sign that it is now permanently devalued" (Lacan, 2006b, p. 280). In essence, lethal alienation denotes that while the subject is deeply entrenched within the system of signifiers, it is simultaneously called to belong to that system. This duality results in the loss and deprivation of the subject's true essence, marking both the point of creation and the moment of disappearance.

To understand lethal alienation more deeply, it is essential to examine Lacan's introduction of the term "aphanisis". Although initially coined by Ernest Jones,

Lacan departs from Jones's original definition, which described it as the fear of losing desire. Instead, Lacan redefines aphanisis to indicate that the subject must be understood in a more profound way, specifically as one who experiences a movement of disappearance, which he refers to as lethal. He describes this phenomenon as the "fading of the subject" (Lacan, 1986g, pp. 207–208). Through the lens of aphanisis, lethal alienation extends beyond a mere dependence between the subject and the Other within the symbolic order. It highlights how the symbolic order generates deprivation and leads to the loss of the subject's substantive core, which, according to philosophical assumptions, is inherently tied to the truth. In the scenario of the "fading of the subject", as noted by Lacan in his discussion of lethal alienation, the Other and the entire field of signifiers impose a lethal factor on the subject. This factor contributes to the ontological castration of the subject's truth. Consequently, this phenomenon of the split subject means that the subject, shaped by its interaction with the symbolic order, emerges as the ego – a false representation that strives to replicate an illusion of being that aligns with a fictionalized reality. It is worth noting that in contrast to this false representation lies the ongoing quest for the subject's true essence.

The concept of aphanisis suggests that lethal alienation reveals a symbolic undermining of the subject's true being, correlating with a state preceding excommunication. Lacan himself describes a period during which his life felt reduced to "the object of what is called a deal" for two years. This lethal alienation, as Lacan articulates, pertains to the psychical-mental condition he experienced, stating,

> It has to do with the situation I was in for two years, that of knowing that I was – at the hands of precisely those who, in relation to me, were colleagues or even pupils – the object of what is called a *deal*.
>
> (Lacan, 1986b, p. 4; italics original)

The paradox lies in the fact that Lacan, as an "object of a deal", attempts to negotiate with a prestigious institution.

Lethal alienation operates in this way: the subject, such as Lacan and individuals in general, is shaped through a compromise that allows for a spatial existence in the symbolic order; however, the true essence of the subject is tragically obscured. After his excommunication, Lacan can no longer be seen as an object of the deal. Therefore, lethal alienation not only mirrors Lacan's psyche before his excommunication, but he also manages to transform his depressive state related to this event into a celebrated form of alienation, which is viewed more positively.

The celebrated form of alienation

The celebrated form of alienation can also be described as positive alienation, where the subject not only recognizes what is missing but also finds satisfaction in detaching from the symbolic order. The symbolic system has a metaphor: it represents a reality that is essentially a virtual illusion, leading the subject to misperceive the self. If this symbolic structure depends on such self-misconceptions, and if the reproduction of these misconceptions serves to sustain the symbolic system, then the "myth of the lamella" contrasts this by representing the libido that flows outside the circuit of meaning. The lamella is not akin to love, as love involves the subject seeking a sexual complement. Instead, the lamella represents the singularity of desire that manifests as a living being without reciprocity.

Once the subject is attached to the lamella, it stuns and shocks the symbolic order. As Slavoj Žižek (2022) states, "Alienation is a condition of our freedom, it gives us a breathing space to exercise freedom" (p. 232). This is connected to the notion of alienation, as it compellingly drives the subject to search for the missing part of the self. This missing part enables a new dimension of the self that lies beyond the symbolic order and is embodied within each individual. The lamella is defined by Lacan as "the extra-flat" that moves like an amoeba and can "survive any division" structurally produced by the symbolic order, such as gender binaries. It also concerns the missing part of the self, such as an asexual being, which stands in contrast to these gender binaries (Lacan, 1986c, p. 197). If the subject ultimately encounters this missing part of the self, that part is no longer unreal. Instead, the unreal is described as "the real in a way that eludes us" (Lacan, 1986g, p. 205). This implies that the missing part of the subject eludes and disconnects from the subject due to the constraints of the symbolic order. However, when the subject finally connects with it, the subject, as the lamella, transcends the role imposed by the symbolic order, which highlights a symptom of that very order.

The lamella represents the cry of the subject (Lacan, 1986g, p. 209), which produces a loud noise that is crucial to understanding the concept of celebrated alienation. This celebrated alienation stems from the subject's drive to find the missing part of themselves. Upon reconnecting with that missing part, the subject can begin to form a unique life that stands in contradiction to the symbolic order. Celebrated alienation is fundamentally tied to this process of rediscovery. In this journey, the subject becomes the lamella, whose distinctive beyond-symbolic existence creates a rift within the symbolic order. This occurs because the lamella acts as a mystical signifier, capable of disrupting the entire process of signification within the symbolic order.

This celebrated form of alienation is positive. In fact, this concept of alienation aligns with Lacan's earlier mention of the subject that is related to the *objet a*, in which the Other knows nothing about such mystical subject (Lacan, 2014, pp. 173–174) in Seminar X, *Anxiety*. In the subsequent Seminar XI, *The Four Fundamental Concepts of Psycho-Analysis*, Lacan continues that a mystical subject is a positive alienation. It is not only alienated by the symbolic order, but it also consents to alienate from it. This subject creates a gap in the symbolic order, and as an unsignified signifier, it causes disintegration within that order. Lacan's most notable example of this celebrated alienation and the concept of the lamella is the word "hommelette" (Lacan, 1986c, p. 197). The term "hommelette" serves as Lacan's *lalangue*; it is a mysterious object of language that refers to neither "egg" nor "home". This characteristic of being an unsignified signifier allows it to free itself from the symbolic order, which is the linguistic system. Therefore, the word *hommelette* embodies his celebrated notion of alienation, where he positively rejects conformity with the symbolic order. Through this rejection, his true subject emerges, as he realizes that his subjectivity – reduced to an object engaged in a transaction – is something that "kills" him and, in this sense, castrates his being.

Connecting Lacan's concept of alienation with the notion of separation is insightful, especially in light of Todd McGowan's observation that "subjectivity is always alienated, far from mastering the world. To be a subject is always to relate to one's world from distance" (McGowan, 2024, p. 28). Since its inception, the formation of truth for the subject has relied heavily on language and the symbolic, leading to a displaced identity. Lacan can be seen as a thinker who utilizes Hegel's dialectic to analyze his own idea on alienation, dividing it into two categories: lethal alienation and celebrated alienation. As Lacan transitioned away from his engagement with the anti-Hegelian faction, his psychoanalytic view of the subject began to align with Hegel's concept of "the self-alienated spirit", which Hegel characterizes as subjectivity, activity, and process (Hegel, 1986, p. 294).

This celebrated form of alienation is engendered by Samo Tomšič, who observes that "from Hegel via Marx to Freud, alienation finally comes to name the constitutively unstable structure of the subject and points toward a decentralized space of thinking, a structure in becoming or a structure as becoming" (Tomšič, 2021, p. 133). Thus, Hegel's perspective on alienation is positive and radical, aligning well with Lacan's celebrated form of alienation, as Hegel argues that "this activity and process whereby the substance becomes *actual* is the alienation of the personality, for the self that has absolute significance in its *immediate* experience" (Hegel, 1986, pp. 294–295; italics original). Hegel asserts that the self-alienated spirit represents a disconnection from the foundation of self-consciousness; the authentic subject embodies the negativity of self-consciousness. (Hegel, 1986, p. 294) until the structure of existing reality undertakes mutation or social metamorphosis because of the self-alienated spirit. McGowan (2024) makes this point that "alienation is the source of all human suffering – if we weren't alienated, we wouldn't suffer – but it is also the source of all satisfaction" (p. 8); this argument resonates with Lacan's celebrated form of alienation.

Celebrated alienation is a constructive form of negativity, symbolizing the life energy that emerges from the individual. It signifies a symbolic negation associated with the subject, which embodies a deep form of negativity. Its aim is not only to restore the subject's true essence but also to highlight a fundamental division within the subject created by the symbolic order: the Other. In this context, the subject identifies itself as both a singular signifier and something distinct from the Other. The subject, as the signifier, distinguishes its own dimensionality from that of the Other, aligning with the idea that "the signifier with which one designates the same signifier is evidently not the same signifier as the one with which one designates the other" (Lacan, 1986g, p. 210). To understand separation, the subject's self-assertion and self-expression as the other (*the objet petit a*) can be seen as a signifier that is materially different from the signifier of the Other, which seeks to map and idealize it according to the imaginary ideals of the Other (the ideal ego). Whether situated within or outside the symbolic order of the Other, separation embodies a distinct characteristic of the subject that is provocatively and passionately resistant to a superficial construction of subjectivity rooted in the field of the Other.

Celebrated alienation refers to the concept of separation as it relates to the subject in a way that demonstrates the principle of dialectic. Separation pertains to the subject that is guided by the dialectic (Lacan, 1986g, p. 213). In this "Hegelian moment", the subject becomes an essential entity of its own, leading Lacan to state, "I shall call it – *separation*" (Lacan, 1986g, p. 213; italics originals). While lethal alienation is the realm of the Other in which the subject chooses to exist and acquire being in the signifier, the separation that embodies celebrated alienation indicates a lack within the discourse of the Other. The separation noted by Lacan aligns with McGowan's observation that separation is constructive as "it frees the subject to experience alienation that defines it as a speaking being by making evident the distance that separates the subject from that identity that purports to define the subject (McGowan, 2024, p. 44). In other words, the philosophical and psychoanalytic argument regarding the subject will ultimately fail unless the subject starts to accept a self-division against the process of symbolic individuation that defines the subject. This event of self-division represents a phenomenology of the self that illustrates the impossibility of achieving objectivity in developing a relationship with the self, while also indicating that the alienation experienced by the individual and their disavowal of the Other contribute to the emergence of the subject. This subject embodies a purity and an excess of being that resonates with Lacan's concept of celebrated alienation, as well as the idea of separation discussed in Seminar XI. In this context, the metonymy of separation including a celebrated form of alienation is represented by terms such as "ferret" (Lacan, 1986g, p. 214) and "amoeba" (Lacan, 1986c, p. 197), which "crawls, slips, escapes" (Lacan, 1986g, p. 214) from the realm of the signifier known as the Other.

Alienation as the proletariat's existence

Understanding Marx's alienation: proletariat and the commodity fetishism

Marx's concept of alienation is primarily discussed in *Capital Volume 1* and the *Economic and Philosophic Manuscripts of 1844*. To fully understand Marx's ideas on alienation, it is essential to examine these two works. Generally, Marx sees alienation as an inherent aspect of the proletariat's existence within the capitalist system of production. He defines alienation as a condition rooted in capitalism, where the proletariat, representing the labor force, experiences a disconnection from their true essence. Understanding alienation cannot be done without considering the proletariat's precarious condition and the dynamics of production. The relation of production creates a cycle that compels the proletariat to repeat their labor time and labor force in order to generate commodities, both quantitatively and qualitatively. This repetition within the social relation of production results in the proletariat's alienation, which is an unavoidable consequence of their circumstances.

In *Capital Volume 1*, Marx's concept of alienation describes the condition of the proletariat in relation to capitalism. Alienation signifies the state of the proletariat within the field of production. It contrasts with the idea of abstract labor, which represents a form of labor that exists outside of the realm of the means of production. Generally, abstract labor cannot exist as alienation. In other words, alienation cannot be equated with the identity of abstract labor. According to Marx, abstract labor refers to human labor that lacks use-value. It describes "the disappearance of the useful character of the products of labor" (Marx, 1990, p. 128). This concept suggests that as long as abstract labor is separated from the social relations of production, it cannot be equated with alienation. Abstract labor cannot express its existence unless it is realized as concrete labor within the social mode of production; it is only in this way that abstract labor can manifest itself (Marx, 1990, p. 150).

Marx's concept of alienation reflects the condition of the proletariat in relation to capitalism and is closely linked to the economic theory of use-value. Use-value refers to the utility of a commodity, with the proletariat being the producer. Marx defines use-value as the usefulness of a commodity – essentially, its utility (Marx, 1990, p. 137). He further states, "The usefulness of a thing makes it a use-value. But this usefulness does not dangle in the mid-air. It is conditioned by the physical properties of the commodity, and has no existence apart from the latter" (Marx, 1990, p. 126). However, the existence of commodities is dependent on the existence of the proletariat. The utility of commodities is tied to the social relations of production, and it is the proletariat that embodies the successful utility of commodities (Edwards and Leiter, 2025, p. 42). The issue arises when the proletariat sees alienation as a normal state of existence rather than making an effort to understand and challenge this oppressive capitalist condition. This misunderstanding is linked to the ideological structures of capitalism, leading the proletariat to accept and sometimes even find comfort in this form of repression (Žižek, 2022, p. 33). As a result, the proletariat's existence is defined by a disconnection from a deeper truth about themselves, leading them to accept alienation as their ordinary reality.

In *Capital Volume 1*, it is noted that alienation reflects the existence of the proletariat. They are separated from the essence of being human, becoming merely a means of adding value to commodities. Alienation characterizes the life of the proletariat, who is immersed in the intense realm of commodity production. This alienation represents an objective condition that poses a challenge to philosophy. The alienation experienced by the proletariat is linked to the production of commodities. While the true essence or life of the proletariat can be understood as the inner self, the production of commodities is viewed as the external object. The tragedy within capitalist social relations is that the proletariat is compelled to become an external object, prioritizing commodity production over their own essential life as an inner being. Marx explains, "The commodity is, first of all, an external object, a thing which through its qualities satisfies human needs of whatever kind" (Marx, 1990, p. 125).

Marx's critique of capitalism suggests that the realm of commodity production serves as a void in the existence of the proletariat. However, Marx also critiques the proletariat for seemingly embracing it. Both their bodies and minds are conditioned to engage with commodity production and are even instrumentalized within capitalist ideology. The use-value of commodities becomes abstract, unless human labor is objectified and is recognized within the social relations of production. According to Marx's concept of alienation, "a use-value, or useful article, therefore, has value only because abstract human labor is objectified or materialized in it" (Marx, 1990, p. 129). This situation threatens proletariat as a philosophical being. Proletariats find themselves trapped in the repetitive cycle of capitalist production, unable to awaken to deeper philosophical questions about their own existence. Marx solves this situation by arguing that philosophy, viewed not merely as an interpretation of history but as a historical evolution, can elevate the spirit of the proletariat.

The analysis of alienation contributes to the concept of "commodity fetishism", as discussed in *Capital Volume 1*. Commodity fetishism is not centered on the production of commodities, nor does it represent merely the enjoyment of consumption and distribution of products. Instead, it highlights how the proletariat reifies themselves within the social relations of production. In this reification, proletariats tend to transform themselves from human beings into objectified commodities in order to produce other commodities, as noted by Georg Lukács (1968, pp. 83–87). Commodity fetishism is closely linked to the material existence of the proletariat. It addresses not the quality or quantity of products but rather emphasizes the exhaustive, and often surplus, labor power and labor time that are embodied in the product.

The condition of the proletariat's existence is closely linked to the concept of commodity fetishism. Marx explains that commodity fetishism reflects not the price and value of the commodity but "the social characteristics of men's own labor as objective characteristics of the products of labor themselves, as the socio-natural properties of these things" (Marx, 1990, pp. 164–165). This also suggests that industrial products are the result of the proletariat, who are not only working in various industrial sectors but are also divided by capitalists into different roles to facilitate commodity production according to their specific skills. Moreover, commodity fetishism does not emphasize the use-value of a commodity (Marx, 1990, p. 164). Instead, it highlights the precarious existence of the proletariat, which is impacted by the objectification of their labor power and labor time. Consequently, "the sum total of the labor of all these private individuals forms the aggregate labor of society" (Marx, 1990, p. 165). Commodity fetishism does not merely reflect the market relationship between demand and supply; it also reveals the historical subjectivity of the proletariat, which is connected to their reification. In the historical context of capitalism, the reification of the proletariat means that they are voluntarily divided based on skill sets and industrial sectors, which reinforces a dominant mode of social production.

In the *Economic and Philosophic Manuscripts of 1844*, Marx conceptualizes alienation in relation to the proletariat's existence as a commodification of labor power. He emphasizes that "the worker sinks to the level of a commodity and becomes indeed the most wretched of commodities" (Marx, 1988a, p. 69). From a critical perspective, Marx defines the proletariat as those who do not possess any means of production. As a result, the proletariat is unable to accumulate wealth or profit. Additionally, it is important to note that Marx critiques the proletariat for making a choice to sacrifice their human freedom – through the process of self-objectification and reification – thereby becoming commodities that produce other commodities.

Marx interprets the proletariat as the working class that paradoxically chooses to reproduce their existence as objectified commodities in order to generate additional commodities. This idea, highlighted in the *Economic and Philosophic Manuscripts of 1844*, is consistent with his arguments in *Capital Volume 1*. He emphasizes that the proletariat's labor and time do not merely produce commodities; the proletariat also produces themselves as a commodity (Marx, 1988a, p. 71). What a commodity seeks to express is not only its price and use-value; instead, it embodies the existence of the proletariat, whose labor power is alienated within that object. Alienation becomes a key concept that defines the existence of the proletariat, as they actively engage in "the objectification of labor" (Marx, 1988a, p. 71) that is reflected in themselves. This may seem paradoxical, but alienation represents a choice made by the proletariat to exist in a state of "object bondage" (Marx, 1988a, p. 71). This is not a manifestation of the proletariat's will to power; rather, it reveals their inclination to accept a position of enslavement within the social relations of production: Marx clearly observes this troubling tendency.

In the *Economic and Philosophic Manuscripts of 1844*, Marx uses the terms "alienation" and "estrangement" interchangeably. While alienation refers to the proletariat's existence and the loss of substantive truth in their social relations of production, estrangement is associated with the idea of the proletariat's political revolution. This connection holds some validity because Marx states that "from the relationship of estranged labor to private property, it follows that the emancipation of society from private property and servitude is expressed in the political form of the emancipation of the workers" (Marx, 1988a, p. 82). However, equating estrangement immediately with the emancipation of the proletariat is somewhat hasty and unconvincing. In other contexts, Marx uses estrangement in the same way as alienation, highlighting that both terms commonly refer to a "loss of reality" (Marx, 1988a, p. 71).

The term "alienation" originates from the German word *entäussern,* which means "to renounce", "to part with", or "to cast off". Its noun form, *entäusserung*, refers to the loss of the inherent essence of something to an external reality. This situation leads to a loss of reality concerning the nature of human being as an existential being. This concept is also closely related to estrangement. To understand estrangement, Marx clearly highlights the proletariat as an instance of estranged labor (Marx, 1988a, p. 69). By this, Marx distinguishes between humans as "species-being" and humans as a "means of individual life" (Marx, 1988a, p. 76). Marx describes humans as "species-being" by referring to them as true beings in themselves, embodying spiritual and communal qualities (Marx, 1988a, pp. 76–77). However, in capitalist society, human beings are reduced to being an estranged labor force, existing primarily as means of individual survival as well as a means of individual life. This existence, rooted in capitalism, erases the essence of humans as species-being. Instead, individuals as a means of survival for others are treated as mere life-activities (Marx, 1988a, p. 76). This situation embodies the essence of estrangement. These life-activities do not clearly promote political emancipation. Rather, they reflect a reality in which all lives are existentially shaped by the social relations of production, perpetuating the cycle of capitalism.

A comparison between Lacan and Marx: an affinity

In order to reexamine Marx's alienation through Lacan's vel of alienation, it is important to explore the affinities and antagonism between Lacan and Marx. To begin with, Marx's concept of alienation addresses the existence of the proletariat, highlighting their depiction as merely a labor force within the social mode of production. As a result, this perspective leads to a loss of the proletariat's intrinsic truth. In comparison, Marx's understanding of alienation is connected to Lacan's notion of lethal alienation, as previously mentioned.

Marx's concept of the proletariat is linked with Lacan's understanding of alienation, which he describes as the object of the deal. This idea suggests that the proletariat makes a rational compromise with capitalism – essentially, the desire of the Other – while simultaneously losing its essence within the realm of the Other. In this sense, negative alienation relates directly to a specific condition of political economy: Lacan's notion of the field of the Other, which he associates with capitalism. This system leads to the erasure of the proletariat's authentic existence. One potential interpretation of the proletariat's speculative truth is that they consciously choose to surrender their identities within the social mode of production. Therefore, the proletariat's existence in a capitalist context signifies a fundamental loss of their inherent truth.

As mentioned earlier, Marx's concept of alienation is closely linked to commodity fetishism. Commodity fetishism highlights how the labor time and force of the proletariat become embodied in commodities, reflecting a historical subjectivism of the proletariat related to their active life-form of self-reification. At this point, Marx's idea of commodity fetishism ties harmoniously with Lacan's notion of lethal alienation. In Lacanian terms, commodity fetishism represents the desire for the Other: specifically, the desire for capitalism as the Other. This demonstrates how the proletariat's existence is deeply rooted in the desire for the Other. Therefore, it is not just the proletariat as individuals who exist, but rather, the existence of capitalism itself is sustained through the repetitive labor and time of the proletariat. The choices made by the proletariat contribute to the ongoing cycle of commodity fetishism. This situation reflects Lacan's exploration of lethal alienation. Within this framework, the proletariat functions as a human resource embedded in the social mode of production, yet they are fated to experience a kind of petrification of their own existence, inevitably.

The psychoanalytic term "aphanisis" refers to an interpretation in which the existence of the proletariat is actively diminished in relation to the Other, particularly within a capitalist mode of production. This concept is connected to Lacan's well-known assertion about the subject: the subject exists in a state of tension with the Other, which is defined as "something that emerges more or less as an identification" (Lacan, 2017, pp. 371–372). The desire of the Other is the external cause that compels the subject to descend into the realm of fantasy, in which the subject becomes obsessional neurosis (Lacan, 2017, p. 369). The subject relates to the object that is nurtured by the Other: the field of fantasy. This suggests that the Other undermines the substantive truth of the subject, transforming the subject from an entity in itself to a subject for the Other, leading to the subject's disappearance or fading. At this juncture, one can observe a parallel between Lacan and Marx. Marx views the existence of the proletariat as analogous to Lacan's fading subject. In the context of commodity fetishism, the proletariat is not simply abstract labor; rather, they embody the material form of labor time and labor power. This attachment is evident in the products they create, as it becomes inseparable from the process of commodity production (Marx,

1990, p. 165). Enthusiastically, it is the proletariat that chooses to be the object of a transactional compromise with capitalism. Marx critiques the existence of the proletariat, stating, "As the foregoing analysis has already demonstrated, this fetishism of the world of commodities arises from the peculiar social character of the labor which produces them" (Marx, 1990, p. 165). From a Lacanian perspective, commodity fetishism embodies the desire of capitalism as the Other, which converts the proletariat from an entity in itself to another signifier, existing for the Other – that is, their existence is subordinated to the demands of commodity fetishism. Thus, this dimension of Marx's political economy, as promoted by Marx himself and traditional Marxism, is intertwined with Lacan's notion of lethal alienation.

However, as mentioned in the introductory chapter, it is insufficient for the proletariat discourse to favor the affinity between Lacan and Marx. It is essential to investigate the contradictions or antagonisms that exist between their ideas. The goal is to consider Lacan as a thinker who introduces a symptom to Marx's understanding of the proletariat.

A contradiction between Lacan and Marx: an antagonism

The concept of existence relates to the proletariat's understanding of the world, which aims to distance itself from and ultimately transform it. From Lacan's perspective, existence can be viewed as *ex-sistence*, representing a form of existence that is invisible and fades into the background of being. If philosophy is fundamentally about critically examining the state of social relations, Lacan's idea of *ex-sistence* ties into the principle of separation, leading to the emergence of a material form of the subject rather than mere idealism. Idealism describes the relationship between the subject and the Other, indicating a state of suspended existence – the loss of the material embodiment of the subject. Lacan connects this material form of the subject to a reversal in the relationship between the subject and the Other (Lacan, 1986g, p. 206). Therefore, in philosophical terms, psychoanalysis distinguishes itself by not treating the existential subject as simply pure idealism. Instead, it is intricately linked to the materialism of the existential subject. This materialism emerges when individuals begin to question their surrounding reality and seek to separate from it, which opens up the possibility for changing the ongoing historical reality.

It is important to highlight the contrast between Lacan's concept of alienation and Marx's focus on the same idea. According to Lacan, alienation is inherently linked to separation. He sees it as a concept that embodies both deviation and detachment from one's surroundings, ultimately containing a sense of liberation. In contrast, Marx emphasizes the need to overcome alienation, which indicates that he interprets alienation without acknowledging any aspect of liberation. Marx's perspective on alienation is closely tied to the idea of commodity fetishism, where the proletariat is trapped within the social mode of production and the objectification of labor. By advocating for the overcoming of alienation, Marx implies a dismissal of the potential to view alienation in a more liberatory context. In brief, Lacan views alienation as a potential source of separation and liberation, whereas Marx perceives it negatively, lacking a liberatory perspective.

Reinterpreting Marx's concept of the proletariat through a Lacanian psychoanalytic lens reveals a discrepancy in their views on alienation. This difference offers a reimagining of Marx's proletariat – an aspect that Marx himself often overlooked. Marx describes the proletariat in relation to alienation as a condition of individual life – specifically, as an estrangement experienced through labor under capitalism. In this context, human beings are reduced to mere assets that sustain commodity fetishism, ultimately leading to a loss of reality for the proletariat. Marx also asserts that "economic estrangement is that of real life" (Marx, 1988b, p. 103). It is explicit that Marx's concept of estrangement lacks a revolutionary quality. By negating religious determinism, Marx highlights class consciousness as authentic life; he argues that overcoming alienation is essential for achieving universal emancipatory politics (Marx, 1988b, pp. 103–104). In contrast, Lacan's notion of alienation posits that striving to overcome alienation is misguided. According to Lacan, the proletariat can emancipate themselves from capitalism not by viewing alienation as an adversary but by recognizing it as a positive form of thought.

Rather than seeking to overcome alienation, the proletariat can embrace it positively. Lacan's reinterpretation of Marx's concept of the proletariat presents proletariat as the myth of the lamella. In this context, the proletariat exists outside the realm of objectification related to their labor forces and labor times. Instead of viewing alienation as a painful condition, the proletariat cultivates an extraordinary space for mutual practice, language, communication, care, empathy, and activity – elements that are foreign to the capitalist Other entangled in commodity fetishism, as discussed in the previous section. This assembly of the proletariat signifies an indefinable space that contrasts sharply with the reduction of proletariat to mere commodity fetishism.

In this ex-capitalist space, the proletariat agrees to embrace alienation. This environment has not yet achieved a new society beyond capitalism. In other words, while this space is shared by the proletariat, it still contrasts with the true form of communism. However, this setting is worth discussing because of its philosophical implications regarding the existence of the proletariat. It resembles what Lacan describes as "amoeba-like", where this proletariat's existence separates from the language of the Other, which is capitalism. This separation allows the proletariat to reformulate their extraordinary existential experiences, leading to new theories, fresh channels of communication, and alternative interpretations of Marxism. It encourages the organization of events that foster care and empathy among themselves. It is important to note that this celebrated form of alienation, practiced by the proletariat, allows them to reinterpret capitalism as a surrounding entity to create distance from it. This perspective is valuable for understanding the proletariat's philosophy of existence. However, it does not imply that revolution has been achieved or that a universal communist utopia has been realized. Even if a communist utopia is achieved, it does not guarantee that the proletariat will not experience alienation. If this occurs, the proletariat may embrace a celebrated form of alienation, finding an alternative to Marx's original vision of communism. The key takeaway is that the proletariat's existence can be likened to a ferret attempting to escape the maze of capital, albeit temporarily, but at risk of returning to the same maze.

This Lacanian reinterpretation of Marx's concept of the proletariat introduces a limitation to Marx's understanding of alienation, which is typically viewed in a negative light. According to Lacan's perspective, the proletariat transitions from being merely the object of capitalist exchanges to actively embracing alienation. This form of alienation reflects the existential condition of the proletariat as a positive negativity, making a significant impact on the realm of the Other, namely capitalism. It is important to recognize that the space beyond capitalism is created by the proletariat, who feel a sense of unbelonging to capitalist ideology. However, this space is still distant from achieving a true emancipatory goal, such as the attainment of a communist society.

The subject of the proletariat: the contradictory principles of the unconscious

The contradictory principles of the unconscious

Understanding the psychoanalytic concept of the unconscious, particularly how it operates within a subject's mental state, requires an examination of its historical development, as a priori.

In the 1920s, the concept of the unconscious was explored in Sigmund Freud's important work, "The Conscious and the Unconscious". In this work, Freud emphasizes that psychoanalysis must acknowledge "the division of the psychic realm into the conscious and the unconscious" (Freud, 2003a, p. 105). He connects the unconscious to the theory of repression, stating, "We thus derive our concept of the unconscious from the theory of repression. The repressed is on our view the paradigm for the unconscious" (Freud, 2003a, p. 107). Repression is linked to the subject's experience of unfulfilled gratification, which Freud describes as an endless "postponement of gratification" (Freud, 2003b, p. 48). To compensate for this loss of satisfaction, the unconscious enables the subject to develop drive-impulses associated with their compulsions, as Freud explains that "the compulsion to repeat is attributable to the unconscious" (Freud, 2003b, p. 58). Consequently, the subject tends to repeat the same actions until they achieve gratification, and repression is thought to be overcome.

In the 1960s, Lacan revisited Freud's concept of the unconscious. In the work "Positions of the Unconscious", Lacan's reinterpretation of Freud allows the unconscious to gain conceptual dynamism, leading to the revelation of contradictory principles within it. More specifically, Lacan's notion of the subject is defined by a fundamental split (*Spaltung*) between the ego and the unconscious (Lacan, 2006a, pp. 708–709). This raises the possibility of understanding the complexities within the unconscious that Lacan himself highlights. In traditional Freudian psychoanalysis, the interpretation of *Spaltung* is fairly conventional. It presents the subject as experiencing internal tension between the ego, which is conscious, and the repressed, which resides in the unconscious. Freud faces criticism here, as his theoretical framework does not sufficiently liberate human desire from social regulation; his understanding of desire is seen as restrictive rather than liberating. In response, the French philosophers Gilles Deleuze and Félix Guattari challenge Freud's assertion about the tension within the subject. Deleuze and Guattari aim to move beyond Freud's psychoanalysis by introducing concepts like "desiring-machines", "the line of flight" from the specific spaces, and "anti-Oedipus schizophrenia", which allow for a more fluid and liberatory conception of desire (Deleuze and Guattari, 2004, pp. 1–54).

Essentially, Lacan's approach differs from those of these two thinkers. While Deleuze's and Guattari's departures from Freud carry significant philosophical and political implications, they does not fully explore the potential to reexamine and redefine the unconscious by allowing it to encompass a Hegelian dialectical imperative. In contrast to the schizophrenic form of unconscious involved with a flow of desire without dialectics, Lacan seeks to alter the meaning of the unconscious as presented by Freud by encompassing Hegelian dialectical imperative. The result of Lacan's employment of Hegelian dialectics to engage with Freud's work is the emergence of contradictory principles within the unconscious as experienced by the subject.

One can explore Lacan's works in greater depth. According to Lacan, the unconscious has three main characteristics. First, accessing the unconscious is impossible without relying on language, as Lacan generalizes that "the unconscious itself has in the end no other structure than the structure of language" (Lacan, 2008b, p. 38). This means that the language used by the subject – whether in the form of a spoken sentence or an intended message – requires careful interpretation by the listener. This enunciated message is necessary to uncover the subject's – speaker's – true thoughts and intentions as the one enunciating the message. The locus of the subject's true thoughts is the Thing (*Das Ding*), which represents itself as the law (Lacan, 2008a, p. 89). Second, language is considered a valuable tool for connecting to the unconscious. The subject's uses of metaphor and metonym allow psychoanalysts to uncover the subject's deepest thoughts, which the subject may be unaware of. Lacan characterizes the unconscious as an active realm of thought that the subject does not realize they know – referred to as the "unknown-known". The third characteristic, which is often overlooked, is the concept of *Spaltung* within the unconscious. This indicates that while the first two characteristics are primary, it is also important to recognize that the unconscious can be divided into two parts: *the Spaltung* in the unconscious itself. Lacan discusses this division of the unconscious in his Seminar V, *Formations of the Unconscious* (1957–1958). He notes that "we know that there is always a *Spaltung*, that is, there are always two lines along which he is constituted" (Lacan, 2017, p. 373). This suggests that it is inevitable for the subject to experience these two lines within the unconscious. The unconscious serves as a source of tension and contradiction for the subject.

For example, consider a subject who experiences the Oedipus complex. The unconscious, functioning as a mental apparatus, can compel the subject, such as an infant, to resent the father, viewing him as an object of envy. Conversely, on another occasion, the same unconscious forces might compel the subject to admire and respect the father, who is perceived as a figure of narcissism and a mature prototype developed within the subject. Consequently, the unconscious contributes to a complex and ambivalent relationship with the father, simultaneously provoking feelings of envy and admiration. This indicates that the unconscious can lead the subject to both despise and idolize the father at the same time.

Lacan's concept of "two lines" refers to the division of the unconscious into two paradoxical functions, which the subject inevitably experiences. This idea highlights an ontology of the subject, suggesting that the individual is compelled by the unconscious to be both compatible and incompatible with social norms simultaneously.

In the first line, the unconscious is connected to the subject by influencing the subject to conform to existing social norms. In other words, the subject remains complicit in these norms because the unconscious drives them to maintain their position without challenging societal expectations. In the second line, which is connected to the first, the unconscious may also push the subject to rebel against society. The psychoanalyst later discovers that the subject exhibits feelings of aggression, envy, hate, violence, lust, and a new perspective on society. This behavior arises because the unconscious operates as a mental apparatus, compelling the subject to think and express themselves in this way. This interplay represents the essence of the unconscious as it manifests in the singularity of the subject.

It is from the second line of thought that the unconscious has the ability to pull the subject back to the first line of thought, preventing them from contemplating social resistance. This creates a cycle where the subject oscillates between the first line and the second line repeatedly. Because of the unconscious, this continuous back-and-forth can generate tension and lead to a self-contradiction within the subject. Lacan suggests that the paradoxical function of the unconscious plays a significant role in shaping the subject. He states, "The dialectic of the subject qua subject of the unconscious" (Lacan, 1986d, p. 242) and emphasizes that "the subject, the Cartesian subject, is what is supposed by the unconscious" (Lacan, 2006a, p. 712). In "Position of the Unconscious", Lacan affirms the paradoxical nature of the unconscious in relation to the formation of the subject. He explains that the subject is connected to the unconscious, noting that "the unconscious is, between two of them, their cut in action" (Lacan, 2006a, p. 712). Furthermore, in *The Four Fundamental Concepts of Psychoanalysis*, Lacan elaborates on these ideas, indicating the complex interplay between the subject and the unconscious:

> This is why such considerations are particularly necessary when it is a question of the unconscious, which I represent to you as that which is inside the subject, but which can be realized only outside, that is to say, in the locus of the Other in which alone it may assume its status.
>
> (Lacan, 1986a, p. 147)

In contrast to Deleuze's concept of a line of flight, in which unconscious is assumedly rhizomatic, and which is deprived of the influence of Hegelian dialectic, Lacan's perspective elucidates that the unconscious is composed of two dialectical lines of thought that represent contradictory principles. These two principles operate from different angles but ultimately converge, akin to a Mobius strip. In relation to the subject, the psychoanalytic principle of *Spaltung* leads to a disunity within the unconscious; there is no unity in this realm. Lacan suggests that the unconscious can be represented cinematically as a montage, where overlapping images and scenes are dialectically antagonistic. Consequently, there are two asymmetrical scenes concerning the unconscious. In the first scene, the subject's unconscious is shaped by the locus of the Other, which includes parents, relatives, the educational system, culture, ideology, the state, and government: the desire of the subject becomes the metaphor of the Other. The subject's unconscious emerges in response to the Other, compelling the subject to repeat behaviors that conform to societal norms, often without any social resistance. This is why Lacan states, in the passage quoted earlier, that unconscious is inside the subject but can be realized only outside, that is to say, in the locus of the Other, in which alone it may assume its status.

However, regarding the principle of *Spaltung* in the unconscious, a more socially rebellious interpretation is required. In the second scene, it is possible that the unconscious compels the subject to resist the locus of the Other. Paradoxically, this leads the subject to become an uncanny Other that disrupts the established norm of the Other. Essentially, the unconscious drives the subject to embody a socially rebellious identity – a subject of resistance. Lacan notes that "the subject receives, from the Other, his own message in the form of unconscious speech. This message, which for him is interdicted, is profoundly misrecognized" (Lacan, 2020, p. 4). This statement indicates the potential of the unconscious to reform and renew the subject, enabling them not to comply with the Other. Because this misrecognition occurs in the context of the Other, Lacan asserts that the unconscious can lead the subject's desires to transcend the locus of the Other. It is through the unconscious that the subject is able to explore a dimension of desire that lies outside the trajectory dictated by the Other. As he expresses it, the subject refers to something "which in the Other as the big Other enables the subject to access this beyond that is to be signified and which is the field we are in the process of exploring, that of his desire" (Lacan, 2017, p. 374). While this may seem rebellious, one should not forget the first scene, which reminds that the unconscious is ontologically contingent. It has the power to curb the subject's behavior, leading them to conform to the norms of the Other, only to resist again, creating a continuous cycle of compliance and rebellion.

Lacan's passage, as quoted earlier, should be read with care. Beyond its original meaning, Lacan also suggests that the unconscious generates a force within the subject that can only be realized externally, as the mysterious Other against the locus of the Other. In this dynamic, the subject, as the mysterious Other, becomes the uncanniness that threatens the Other. But this relationship alone is insufficient. The force of the unconscious can simultaneously position the subject as both compliant and resistant to social norms – like a Mobius strip, where the unconscious functions like a cinematic montage. This contradiction lies at the heart of the principles of the unconscious, which will be used to reinterpret Marx's concept of the proletariat.

The proletariat unconscious

Marx does not address the role of the unconscious in the psychological domain of humans, which reveals limitations in his understanding of the subjectivity of the proletariat. Because he is not a psychoanalyst, Marx can only recognize the proletariat as a working class that collectively endures suffering. His perspective is predominantly economic, defining the proletariat primarily as a labor force instrumentalized in the modes of production that benefit the growth of capitalism. Marx tends to reduce the concept of proletariat to merely the working class, the wage laborers who sacrifices their labor power for the capitalist system in order to live (Marx and Engels, 2004, p. 21). This interpretation overlooks critical psychoanalytical aspects, particularly how the contradictory principles of the unconscious significantly influence the formation of the proletariat's subjectivity.

The contradictory principles of the unconscious are significant in highlighting how the unconscious acts as a powerful force that compels the proletariat to engage with capitalism. On one hand, it drives them to immerse themselves in the capitalist system, while on the other hand, it simultaneously urges them to resist and not submit to capitalism. This extreme and contradictory nature of the unconscious is a primary cause of the internal conflict within the proletariat regarding their ambivalence toward capitalism. Rather than defining the proletariat solely as the working class involved in capitalism, this paradoxical function of the unconscious helps to broaden economic understanding. It contributes to an awareness of what can be called the proletariat unconscious, which characterizes the proletariat as a complex subject.

The first line of the unconscious compels the proletariat to connect their lives to capitalism. This line is a significant cause of a lethal form of alienation. As previously noted, lethal alienation connects to the loss of reality within the realm of commodity fetishism. The key point is that the proletariat does not choose this lethal alienation; rather, it is brought about by the first line of the unconscious that forces the proletariat to continue experiencing this alienation – as an objectification in the mode of production: it is unconscious that chooses this form of alienation for the proletariat. In relation to capitalism, aspects of the proletariat's unconscious, such as libido, sex, lust, and various drives, are sublimated and objectified to fulfill the desires of capitalism. Because the unconscious exerts a powerful influence, it becomes challenging for the proletariat to resist this compulsion. It suppresses any attempt at resistance by shaping their subjectivity to align with capitalist interests and finds ego-satisfaction in the capitalist arena. In other words, the first line of the unconscious compels the proletariat to develop a subjectivity that harmoniously fits within capitalist objectivity. This unconscious force transforms the proletariat into a money-making machine and the debt subjects, keeping them objectified within the social mode of production, even to structurally entrenched in a deep joy of self-proletarianization. Consequently, it leads them to perceive the reality of capitalism as a singular entity, suppressing any potential for social upheaval. The first line of the unconscious generates the effect of lethal alienation until the proletariat's subjectivity is molded to sustain capitalism without fluctuation.

The second line of the unconscious – still connected to the first – refers to a dynamic process that operates in an opposite direction before returning to its original state. This suggests that the unconscious is a force that enables the proletariat to contemplate social change. It forces proletariat to imagine the world beyond capitalism such as the world without money, scarcity, and full of abundance assisted by technology and automation, including the concept of a communist future. Without the direct control of the conscious mind, this imaginative world is launched by the unconscious: it is the repressed desire that enables these imaginative worlds in the subjectivity of the proletariat. This characteristic of the unconscious reveals a power that allows individuals to disavow capitalism as a given reality and to envision a world that transcends the capitalist framework. This dimension of the unconscious empowers the proletariat to escape the influences of the capitalist Other, producing a drive toward social upheaval that reflects their subjective experience. The second line of the unconscious positions the proletariat as a subject that confronts capitalism, creating a unique proletarian universe filled with language and worldviews that resist the dominant symbolic language of capitalism. It is this aspect of the unconscious, which lies beyond the proletariat's conscious control, that articulates a counter-narrative against the pervasive nature of capitalism. The power of the unconscious grants the proletariat the ability to conceive, reflect on, and imagine a post-capitalist world within their own imaginative frameworks. It is assumed that the post-capitalist world envisioned by the proletariat becomes visible precisely because of this second line of the unconscious.

The second line of the unconscious is intricately linked to a celebrated form of alienation. From a psychoanalytical perspective, the communist imaginary expressed by the proletariat can be understood as a compulsion to repeat the contemplation of a world beyond capitalism. This second line of the unconscious enables the proletariat to experiment with crossing the boundary of the existing capitalist principle. It allows them to enter a realm that exists beyond the current frontier of capitalist framework before returning to the familiar conditions of their reality. It is important to understand that the communist imaginary serves as a signifier of the uncanniness present within capitalism. This imaginary is continuously produced by the second line of the unconscious, which can be viewed as a drive that does not belong to any specific individual or group. There exists a communist imaginary generated by this second line of the unconscious for the proletariat, one that is distinct from both capitalism and Marxism. This communist imaginary imposes a sense of uncanniness upon Marx himself. This is why Lacan, following Freud, articulates the drive as "a belonging neither to __ (insert a) nor to __ (insert b)" (Lacan, 2006a, p. 715).

Because of the second line of the unconscious, there is potential to envision a communist imaginary that transcends the signifier of Marxism. This communist imaginary represents the *objet a*, or small o. Its compulsion to repeat such a communist signifier functions similarly to the imagery of "the peacock's feather, the gas-tap goes into the lady's mouth, and the bird's rump emerges in the middle" (Lacan, 1986f, p. 169). This illustrates a signifier of a communist imaginary that goes beyond Marxism. This does not imply that the subject of the proletariat is a non-human entity. Instead, it resonates with Lacan's myth of the lamella, embodied by the proletariat. In other words, there exists an ideal image of post-capitalism driven by the second line of the unconscious, which represents a celebrated form of alienation. This ideal image, enabled by the second line of the unconscious, does not belong to capitalist reality or Marxist theory. However, the proletariat should positively embrace this celebrated form of alienation. As McGowan states, "the unconscious finds satisfaction in creating and sustaining alienation because there is no initial satisfying object. The subject discovers a satisfying object only through a loss that gives the subject something to desire" (McGowan, 2024, p. 20).

Following the law of contradictory principles in the unconscious, the second line of the unconscious – which permits the proletariat's antagonism to capitalism – can be nullified and neutralized by the first line of the unconscious. Consequently, the proletariat may retreat into capitalism, becoming negatively alienated in the realm of commodity fetishism. In this dynamic, the first line of the unconscious reasserts its influence, allowing for a superficially celebrated form of alienation and a return to the original capitalist position. This process resembles a Mobius strip, oscillating back and forth until the proletariat's unconscious experiences its own *Spaltung*, resulting in a significant contradiction within the unconscious. This complexity in the unconscious highlights a deficiency in Marx's framework, which lacks a psychoanalytic perspective regarding the subjectivity of the proletariat.

Politics: overcoming alienation and its discontent

In the introductory chapter, it is noted that Lacan and Marx share a common perspective on resisting capitalism. The main thesis of the proletariat discourse presents a political viewpoint that diverges from both Left populism and the Lacanian Left, which focus on the hegemonic articulation of antagonistic political identities against oppressive regimes while reluctantly accepting anti-capitalism as a universal stance. Marx views the proletariat as a political agent for social revolution, a concept that corresponds with Lacan's notion of exiting capitalism. Marx argues that the proletariat's revolution is essential for overcoming alienation, emphasizing that true liberation from alienation is unattainable without the class consciousness of the proletariat.

The theoretical perspectives of traditional Marxism are often overly optimistic. While Lacan talks about the possibility of removing capitalism from the lives of the collective proletariat, he is primarily focused on the notion of alienation, which is deeply ingrained in the psyche and subjectivity of the proletariat. Psychoanalysis reveals that alienation – both its lethal and celebrated forms – emerges from the internal contradictions within the proletariat due to the paradoxical nature of the unconscious. From a psychoanalytic standpoint, two critical questions arise: How can Marx and traditional Marxism eliminate this sense of alienation from the psyche and subjectivity of the proletariat? Additionally, how can they address the contradictory principles of the unconscious that compel the proletariat to both accept and resist capitalism while relying solely on the obsolete concepts of class consciousness and the overcoming of alienation? The outdated theoretical tools are insufficient to grasp the complex realities of the proletariat and its connection to anti-capitalist politics.

At this point, it is impossible for Marx to regard the proletariat as a political agency without addressing the proletariat's experience of alienation, in which its essence is dialectically converged in a twofold manner. In the first side of alienation, it is a lethal form of alienation. This is compelled by the first line of the unconscious. It tends to determine the proletariat to remain pleased with the objectifications of labor in capitalism. Capitalism relies on the proletariat as a human being whose exercise of freedom in the form of labor force in attaining the utility of things requires an exchange of labor force with wage (Engels, 1988, p. 181). Capitalism is deceitful enough in letting the proletariat misidentify themselves as the human value-asset highly significant in the production process and extensively valuable for the workplace. In psychoanalytic understanding, the proletariat is at risk of gaining pleasure such as a higher salary rate, promotion, and social mobility by unconsciously becoming nothing else but a capitalist's mode of production that relies on the fantasy of meritocracy imposed upon the proletariat. This lethal form of alienation experienced by the proletariat resonates with Lacan's aphanisis, leading to the loss of the proletariat's speculative truth in the field of the capitalist Other. Operated in tandem with Lacan's aphanisis described in *The Four Fundamental Concepts of Psycho-Analysis* as "the subject fades away" because of the effect of the signifier representing not its true being (Lacan, 1986d, p. 236), Marx in *Wages, Price, and Profit* also warns that the proletariat is at risk to see the price or value of his labor force sacrificing his freedom for an expansion of capitalism as the loss of the proletariat true being in itself (Marx and Engels, 2024, p. 111).

In the second side of alienation, there exists a celebrated form of alienation. This is driven by the unconscious's second line, which compels the proletariat to seek social change. The unconscious suddenly prompts the proletariat to adopt an antagonistic position against capitalism, although this stance is temporary as they might revert to the first level of alienation. Nonetheless, this trajectory of the unconscious fosters this celebrated form of alienation, allowing the proletariat to envision a post-capitalist imaginary that transcends the current reality of capitalism. This emergence of the *objet a* – notably the small o – is significant as it represents the communist imaginary that diverges from Marx's discourse on the subject of the proletariat. As mentioned in the previous chapter, *objet a* signifies a form of non-relationship, revealing a discrepancy within the totality of the discourse. This discrepancy indicates that the discourse is merely a semblance of the truth rather than the truth itself. Lacan emphasizes that "there is no subject without, somewhere, an aphanisis of the subject, and it is in this alienation, in this fundamental division, that the dialectic of the subject is established" (Lacan, 1986h, p. 221). Consequently, it is the unconscious that drives the proletariat to resist capitalism, as they adopt a dialectical stance against the disappearance of the self – an aphanisis – in relation to capitalism.

Instead of adhering to traditional Marxist concepts like overcoming alienation and developing class consciousness, the revolutionary movement of the proletariat should recognize the inherently paradoxical nature of the unconscious. It is insufficient to merely overcome alienation; what is politically and psychoanalytically necessary is to confront the vel of alienation and the contradictory principles of the unconscious. The paradoxical nature of the unconscious, as articulated through Lacan's concept of *Spaltung*, suggests that there is no guarantee that a proletariat with class consciousness can consistently engage in revolutionary actions. From a political-psychoanalytic standpoint, this psychoanalytic perspective challenges Lacan's compatibility with Marx. Class consciousness presupposes that the proletariat, in Marxism's analysis, is unaffected by the contradictory dynamics of the unconscious. However, it is precisely the proletariat that possesses class consciousness that embodies a relationship with the unconscious, all while striving to achieve its revolutionary goals, values, and freedoms. Despite having class consciousness, the unconscious can drive proletariats to self-objectify as labor forces and measure their worth in terms of labor time and productivities, ultimately contributing to the perpetuation of capitalism. Overcoming the paradoxical nature of the unconscious is a far greater challenge – if not impossible – than simply overcoming alienation. This Lacanian psychoanalytic critique of Marx's concept of the proletariat presents a challenge to traditional Marxism, urging a reevaluation of revolutionary theory within academic discourse.

To sum up this chapter, Marx's understanding of the proletariat is closely linked to several key concepts, such as commodity fetishism and alienation. His negative perspective on alienation resonates with Lacan's idea of lethal alienation. However, Marx overlooks a potentially positive aspect of alienation, often referred to as celebrated alienation in this chapter. This dimension highlights a fundamental tension between Marx and Lacan. While Marx regards the proletariat as a pivotal political agent in the fight against capitalism, his interpretation of the proletariat's subjectivity has its limitations. He primarily sees the proletariat in terms of a working class that engages in wage labor, exchanging their labor for compensation and investing time into their work. Through a Lacanian reinterpretation of Marx, one can argue that the proletariat grapples with contradictory forces within the unconscious, leading them to both resist capitalism and, paradoxically, conform to it. It seems that the proletariat must choose between two types of alienation. Notably, it suggests that the unconscious drives the proletariat to alternate between resisting capitalism and submitting to it. It is the unconscious that chooses both forms of alienation for the proletariat. This dynamic poses a challenge to traditional Marxist views on class consciousness and overcoming alienation. In relation to the previous chapter, Marx economically frames the proletariat as a working class. In contrast, a Lacanian psychoanalytic perspective allows us to view the proletariat as a hysterical subject. Instead of defining the proletariat solely as the working class, this chapter ultimately shows how the proletariat experiences two forms of alienation, driven by the conflicting principles of the unconscious that shape their subjectivity.

Reference list

Deleuze, G., and Félix Guattari (2004). 'The Desiring-Machines', in *Anti-Oedipus: Capitalism and Schizophrenia*. Translated by Robert Hurley, Mark Seem, and Helen Lane. London and New York: Continuum.

Engels, F. (1988). 'Outlines of a Critique of Political Economy', in *Economic and Philosophic Manuscripts of 1844 and the Communist Manifesto*. Translated by Martin Milligan. New York: Prometheus Books.

Freud, S. (2003a) 'The Conscious and the Unconscious', in *Beyond the Pleasure Principle and Other Writings*. Translated by John Reddick. Introduced by Mark Edmundson. London: Penguin Books.

Freud, S. (2003b). *Beyond the Pleasure Principle and Other Writings*. Translated by John Reddick. Introduced by Mark Edmundson. London: Penguin Books.

Hegel, G. (1977). 'Spirit', in *Phenomenology of Spirit*. Translated by A.V. Miller. Oxford: Oxford University Press.

Lacan, J. (1986a). 'Analysis and the Truth or the Closure of the Unconscious', in *The Seminar of Jacques Lacan Book XI: The Four Fundamental Concepts of Psychoanalysis*. Edited by Jacques-Alain Miller. Translated by Alan Sheridan. London: Penguin Books.

Lacan, J. (1986b). 'Excommunication', in *The Seminar of Jacques Lacan Book XI: The Four Fundamental Concepts of Psychoanalysis*. Edited by Jacques-Alain Miller. Translated by Alan Sheridan. London: Penguin Books.

Lacan, J. (1986c). 'From Love to the Libido', in *The Seminar of Jacques Lacan Book XI: The Four Fundamental Concepts of Psychoanalysis*. Edited by Jacques-Alain Miller. Translated by Alan Sheridan. London: Penguin Books.

Lacan, J. (1986d). 'Of the Subject Who is Supposed to Know, Of the First Dyad, and Of the Good', in *The Seminar of Jacques Lacan Book XI: The Four Fundamental Concepts of Psychoanalysis*. Edited by Jacques-Alain Miller. Translated by Alan Sheridan. London: Penguin Books.

Lacan, J. (1986e). 'Preface to the English-Language Edition', in *The Seminar of Jacques Lacan Book XI: The Four Fundamental Concepts of Psychoanalysis*. Edited by Jacques-Alain Miller. Translated by Alan Sheridan. London: Penguin Books.

Lacan, J. (1986f). 'The Deconstruction of the Drive', in *The Seminar of Jacques Lacan Book XI: The Four Fundamental Concepts of Psychoanalysis*. Edited by Jacques-Alain Miller. Translated by Alan Sheridan. London: Penguin Books.

Lacan, J. (1986g). 'The Subject and the Other: Alienation', in *The Seminar of Jacques Lacan Book XI: The Four Fundamental Concepts of Psychoanalysis*. Edited by Jacques-Alain Miller. Translated by Alan Sheridan. London: Penguin Books.

Lacan, J. (1986h). 'The Subject and the Other: Aphanisis', in *The Seminar of Jacques Lacan Book XI: The Four Fundamental Concepts of Psychoanalysis*. Edited by Jacques-Alain Miller. Translated by Alan Sheridan. London: Penguin Books.

Lacan, J. (2006a). 'Position of the Unconscious', in *Écrits: The First Complete Edition in English*. Translated by Bruce Fink. London and New York: W.W. Norton & Company.

Lacan, J. (2006b). 'Variations on the Standard Treatment', in *Écrits: The First Complete Edition in English*. Translated by Bruce Fink. London and New York: W.W. Norton & Company.

Lacan, J. (2008a). 'On the Moral Law', in *The Seminar of Jacques Lacan Book VII: The Ethics of Psychoanalysis*. Edited by Jacques-Alain Miller. Translated by Dennis Porter. London and New York: Routledge.

Lacan, J. (2008b). 'Pleasure and Reality', in *The Seminar of Jacques Lacan Book VII: The Ethics of Psychoanalysis*. Edited by Jacques-Alain Miller. Translated by Dennis Porter. London and New York: Routledge.

Lacan, J. (2014). 'Aphorisms on Love', in *The Seminar of Jacques Lacan Book X: Anxiety*. Edited by Jacques-Alain Miller. Translated by A.R. Price. Cambridge and Malden: Polity Press.

Lacan, J. (2017). 'The Other's Desire', in *The Seminar of Jacques Lacan Book V: Formations of the Unconscious*. Edited by Jacques-Alain Miller. Translated by Russell Grigg. Cambridge and Maden: Polity Press.

Lacan, J. (2020). 'Introduction', in *The Seminar of Jacques Lacan Book IV: The Object Relation*. Edited by Jacques Alain-Miller. Translated by A.R. Price: Cambridge and Medford: Polity Press.

Lukács, G. (1968). 'Reification and the Consciousness of the Proletariat', in *History and Class Consciousness: Studies in Marxist Dialectics*. Translated by Rodney Livingstone. Cambridge and Massachusetts: The MIT Press.

Marx, K. (1988a). '[Estranged Labor]', in *Economic and Philosophic Manuscripts of 1844 and the Communist Manifesto*. Translated by Martin Milligan. New York: Prometheus Books.

Marx, K. (1988b). '[Private Property and Communism. Various Stages of Development of Communist Views. Crude, Equalitarian Communism and Communism as Socialism Coinciding with Humaneness]', in *Economic and Philosophic Manuscripts of 1844 and the Communist Manifesto*. Translated by Martin Milligan. New York: Prometheus Books.

Marx, K. (1990). 'The Commodity', in *Capital: A Critique of Political Economy Volume 1*. Translated by Ben Fowkes. London and New York: Penguin Classics.

Marx, K., and Friedrich Engels. (2004). 'Manifesto of the Communist Party', in *Essential Thinkers: Karl Marx*. London: CRW Publishing Limited.

Marx, K., and Friedrich Engels. (2024). 'Wage, Price, and Profit', in *The Communist Manifesto & Other Selected Writings*. London: William Collins.

McGowan, T. (2024). *Embracing Alienation: Why We Shouldn't Try to Find Ourselves*. London: Repeater Books.

Schacht, R. (1992). 'Hegel, Marx, Nietzsche, and the Future of Self-Alienation', in *Alienation, Society, and the Individual: Continuity and Change in Theory and Research*. Edited by Felix Geyer, and Walter R. Heinz. New Brunswick and London: Transaction Publishers.

Tomšič, S. (2021). 'Elements of a History of Alienation', in *The Labor of Enjoyment: Towards a Critique of Libidinal Economy*. Berlin: August Verlag.

Žižek, S. (2016). 'From Human to Posthuman . . . And Back to Inhuman: The Persistence of Ontological Difference', in *Disparities*. London and New York: Bloomsbury.

Žižek, S. (2022). 'Surplus-Enjoyment, Or, Why Do We Enjoy Our Oppression', in *Surplus-Enjoyment*. London and New York: Bloomsbury.

5 A dialectic of proletariat self-enjoyment

From a pathological existence to the proletariat in a logic of Lacanian Woman

This chapter emphasizes that Karl Marx's critique of capitalism is connected to enjoyment. Marx's understanding of enjoyment is closely linked to the conditions of the capitalist mode of production. It describes a capitalist class that revels in the accumulation of capital while the proletariat faces collective misery (Marx and Engels, 2004, p. 52), ultimately resulting in structural class warfare. Marx describes capitalism as the material condition that "establishes an accumulation of misery, corresponding with accumulation of capital. Accumulation of wealth at one pole is, therefore, at the same time accumulation of misery, agony of toil, slavery, ignorance, brutality, mental degradation, at the opposite pole" (Marx, 2004, p. 389). In contrast to Marx's understanding of enjoyment, Jacques Lacan's psychoanalytic notion of enjoyment highlights different aspects of enjoyment – masochism, sadism, narcissism, divine enjoyment – that are interconnected with the condition of the proletariat.

This chapter is organized into four sections, each addressing a fundamental dimension of proletariat discourse that was introduced earlier. In the first section, Lacan's authentic understanding of enjoyment is explored, emphasizing that enjoyment is dialectical; it fluctuates among masochism, sadism, and narcissism. This dialectical nature of enjoyment contests the Marxist perspective, which tends to reduce the psychological dimension of the proletariat to mere class consciousness, implying that class consciousness exists without any internal resistance within the proletariat's psychological framework. The second section examines how these three psychoanalytic dimensions of enjoyment contribute to a pathological existence within the proletariat's dialectical self-enjoyment. It discusses masochistic, sadistic, and narcissistic enjoyment as conditions that the proletariat must interpret through philosophy, allowing them to understand their relationship with the pathologized capitalist world before they can enact meaningful change.

The third section explores Lacan's idea of the splitting nature of the subject. This concept introduces the possibility of the proletariat transcending their pathological existence to become a revolutionary subject. This perspective highlights

DOI: 10.4324/9781003657781-5

a form of self-enjoyment among the proletariat that is aligned with the logic of Lacanian concepts of woman and divine enjoyment. This idea of female desire as a divine enjoyment, manifested by the proletariat, is a psychoanalytical aspect that is often overlooked in Marx's depiction of the proletariat as mere workers enduring collective misery, as well as traditional Marxism's focus on class consciousness.

The fourth section posits that the proletariat is a revolutionary agency. It emphasizes the need for the proletariat to embrace what is termed "divine violence", positioning themselves as embodiments of a divine force in their quest for revolutionary change, rather than rejecting the influence of the divine in the political transition from capitalism to communism. However, this perspective must be approached with caution, as it does not account for the inherent ontological gap experienced by the proletariat. There is no guarantee that the proletariat's encounter with divine enjoyment will be sustained; they may well revert to masochistic, sadistic, and narcissistic enjoyment, oscillating between cooperation with capitalism and the pursuit of divine enjoyment and divine violence in their resistance to it – similarly to the movement of a Mobius strip: a merging of two opposing directions makes it impossible to distinguish between the sites of interiority and exteriority.

The three psyches of enjoyment: masochism, sadism, and narcissism

This section highlights Lacan's original conceptualization of enjoyment, which includes three psychoanalytic dimensions: masochism, sadism, and narcissism. These dimensions are valuable for understanding the proletariat and the development of self-enjoyment within them. These dimensions deviate from the general psychology theory, which posits that enjoyment arises from a singular relationship between human good emotions and the satisfying objects, such as enhancing enjoyment for the athlete (McCarthy and Jones, 2005, p. 158). This conventional understanding of enjoyment – referred to as the Gestalt of enjoyment – involves aspects that generate a sense of aesthetics and pleasure, characterized by the inherent attractiveness of an object that both captivates and generates good emotion in the individual. However, when viewed from a Lacanian perspective, the three dimensions of enjoyment become intertwined with the subject's complexity, as well as their uncertainty and ambiguity.

In terms of translation, it is important to note that there is no precise or adequate English translation for Lacan's term *jouissance*, which truly reflects the depth and nuance of his thought. Alan Sheridan, a prominent translator of Lacan's works, points out that while enjoyment may convey some meaning, such as enjoyment of rights or property, the term has lost the sexual connotations that it retains in French. In this context, enjoyment cannot capture the sense of *jouissance* as the latter is interlaced with the impossibility of the sexual relationship and the lack of the formation of a definitive sexual identity. Sheridan further explains that *jouir* is actually a slang term meaning "to come". In contrast, the English word "enjoyment" conveys a rather hollow sense of "to come", which might suggest simply that there is something more "to arrive" (Sheridan as cited in Lacan, 1986, p. 281). If one adheres strictly to Sheridan's suggestion, they should refrain from equating *jouissance* with enjoyment. If one decides to view *jouissance* as a form of enjoyment, it is important to also consider that this enjoyment can involve social transgression and more addiction to repeating the same action, even in the face of social punishment and threats.

In addition, it is a misconception to regard enjoyment merely as an emotional category, such as pleasure, joy, or happiness; instead, Lacan's remarkable understanding of enjoyment is shaped by a Hegelian dialectical procedure that redefines the common perception of enjoyment. To truly understand enjoyment in this psychoanalytical context means recognizing it as indicative of an ontological split within the term itself. This understanding of enjoyment allows one to grasp it in relation to the complexity of human subjects and their psyches. For example, an individual experiences enjoyment in various forms. This particular individual embodies multiple aspects of enjoyment, enabling them to internalize masochistic, sadistic, and narcissistic tendencies in themselves.

At this point, there are two points to note. First, it is observed that Lacan's conceptualization of enjoyment addresses a profound process of self-division and the internal conflicts inherent in this notion. Second, an individual experiences enjoyment in different forms within themselves. Consequently, this radical hypothesis allows for a philosophical and psychoanalytical reexamination of enjoyment, while preventing it from being conflated with human sentimentality, which is tied to singularity or a uniform domain of human emotion promoted by the theory of general psychology. In other words, by following the critical approach offered by Lacanian psychoanalysis and seeking an epistemological reevaluation of the term, enjoyment should be redefined to reflect a dialectical effect – exhibiting a scenario of internal self-dissensus of the term.

This Lacanian interpretation of enjoyment leads to a hypothesis about the proletariat's capacity for self-enjoyment. It highlights an antagonism with Marx's understanding of enjoyment. Given his limited engagement with psychoanalysis, Marx connects enjoyment primarily to the emotional dimension. As a non-psychoanalyst, his conception of enjoyment remains rooted in emotional categories or sentimentality. As mentioned earlier, Marx appears to equate enjoyment with the joy and pleasure of the capitalist, while the proletariat is obstructed from experiencing the same. This is evident when Marx argues that capitalists derive enjoyment, or joy, from their ownership of the means of production and from increased profits, while the proletariat is deprived of such enjoyment. While Marx acknowledges the relationship between capitalism and enjoyment, he tends to overlook the proletariat's potential for self-enjoyment. Reinterpreting Marx's views on the proletariat aims to demonstrate that this self-enjoyment is ontologically dialectical: the dialectic of the proletariat's self-enjoyment. On the one hand, it represents a form of self-enjoyment enacted by the proletariat that sustains capitalism, and on the other, it encompasses a type of self-enjoyment that threatens capitalism. This dialectical form of enjoyment inherent in the proletariat is something Marx fails to recognize in his understanding of them.

Traditional Marxism emphasizes a theory of class consciousness; however, it tends to overlook the dimension of self-contradiction or the dialectic within the proletariat's self-enjoyment. Developing from Lacan's original insights, it is possible to identify three psychoanalytic dimensions of enjoyment embodied by the proletariat that contribute to the continuity of capitalism. First, masochistic enjoyment refers to the pleasure the proletariat derives from acquiring an object that ultimately betrays their true desires. Despite this betrayal, the proletariat often pretends to enjoy the object, becoming almost addicted to it, as if it fulfills their genuine desires. This form of enjoyment prevents them from seeking out objects that could actually satisfy their true desires. Second, sadistic enjoyment is associated with the proletariat's actions that harm others, such as bullying colleagues and deeply engaging in the dirty game of office politics. This enjoyment derived from the violation of others becomes an addictive behavior, which hinders the possibility of genuine political action aimed at overthrowing capitalism. Third, narcissistic enjoyment pertains to those members of the proletariat who have succeeded within capitalism and own means of production. However, this form of ownership can lead to a tragic cycle of exploitation, reflecting the complex nature of their success. It is important to note that these three dimensions of enjoyment are not separate categories; rather, a single proletariat can embody all forms of enjoyment simultaneously. Ultimately, these three theses on proletariat's self-enjoyment demonstrate the pathological existence of the proletariat that contributes to a continuity of capitalism.

The pathological existence of the proletariat and the continuity of capitalism

Masochistic enjoyment

The first pathological existence of the proletariat is masochistic enjoyment. This idea is derived from Lacan, who insists that the fundamental principle of enjoyment is centered on pleasure, which is intertwined with pain, indicating that desire stems from a lack of satisfaction, and that it is ultimately unattainable, yet the subject continues to seek the cause of this desire (Lacan, 1999c, p. 6). This does not mean that individuals experience a lack of fulfillment or satisfaction, nor does it imply that desire is temporary. Pleasure can be successfully achieved, and the source of that pleasure appears to satisfy the subject's desires and enables the subject to preserve life. However, this satisfaction can lead to feelings of betrayal, as the object ultimately fails to provide true fulfillment. This means that the object of enjoyment that represents an object presence-at-hand ultimately proves to be misaligned with the subject's deeper desires. Masochistic enjoyment occurs when the subject "takes on the position of loss or waste represented by *a* at the level of surplus jouissance" (Lacan, 2024b, p. 113). According to Lacan, at the level when the subject derives surplus-enjoyment, the subject still feels the loss or waste in relation to the object that gives them a surplus-enjoyment. This feeling of loss and waste leads to feelings of betrayal. But the object of betrayal transforms into a fetish that the individual fantasizes to align with their desires. Unlike a lack, which involves a continual craving for more, betrayal stems from unmet expectations of fulfillment. Despite this, the individual still feels compelled to embrace the object of betrayal as if it were genuine satisfaction; otherwise, the enjoyment derived from it will completely disappear. This is the origin of masochism, which involves a person's willingness to continue living with a form of pleasure that is mixed with pain connected to the object of that pleasure – a pleasure derived from pain.

In Lacan's seminar titled *The Object Relation*, he suggests that the object of enjoyment is inherently deceptive, as it cannot be seen as a harmonious entity that connects the subject with reality or the subject's true desires. The phobia object and the fetish object generate a strange form of enjoyment in the subject. Lacan argues that the ontological nature of those objects is imaginary object: "the object is not regarded in the same terms as in the new-fangled theory, a fully satisfying object, the object par excellence, a harmonious object, the object that grounds man in a corresponding reality" (Lacan, 2021, p. 7). In addition, the history of psychoanalysis supports Lacan's conceptualization of enjoyment. This concept relates to the idea that pleasure often comes intertwined with pain and betrayal, a theme discussed for decades in Sigmund Freud's notion of object-love. In *Beyond the Pleasure Principle*, Freud argues that the subject's possession of the love object, such as the mother's breast during the oral stage, is simultaneously associated with feelings of hate and anxiety (Freud, 2003, p. 93). In this context, it is misleading to blame external factors alone, such as the Oedipal father, who possesses the mother and acts as a repressive force regarding the castration of desire. The father symbolizes the cause of separation between the mother and the subject, in this case, the children. In a typical Freudian manner, enjoyment is not merely tied to the Oedipal father as the sole source of guilt and shame; rather, it stems from an enjoyment related to the mother's body, which inherently produces an "ambivalence of love and hate" (Freud, 2003, p. 94). The essence of masochism is that the subject grapples with enjoying this flawed aspect and must embrace it, maintaining it as the true source of pleasure to avoid losing the entirety of that enjoyment.

How does the psychoanalytic aspect of masochism contribute to the proletariat's self-masochistic enjoyment, an aspect that Marx overlooks? Rather than viewing capitalism as a source of betrayal that generates both pain and pleasure for the proletariat, Marx sees it purely as a system of social production determined by economic relationships. He describes these relationships in terms of raw materials, instruments of labor, and various means of subsistence, aiming to solidify all aspects of social relations governed by the logic of capitalist economic production (Marx, 2024, p. 71). However, Marx's recognition shows a negligence of a Lacanian psychoanalytic perspective in twofold. First, in his understanding of the proletariat, Marx fails to recognize a masochistic form of enjoyment that enables the proletariat to endure capitalism without acknowledging their misery. Second, Marx's analysis also overlooks that capitalism embodies a structural reality of desire, lack, and fantasy. While he brilliantly acknowledges capitalism as a socio-economic relationship, psychoanalysis posits that capitalism functions as a phantasmatic system of desire capable of fulfilling a lack. It presents itself as the Other, operating on a principle of meritocracy, and ultimately offers the object of desire that the proletariat seeks to fulfill within capitalism, until their revolutionary impulses are eventually repressed.

The current stage of capitalism operates alongside meritocracy. This ideology, which is intricately organized by the middle class, offers individuals with exceptional abilities the opportunity for social mobility within the capitalist system (Young, 2008, p. 142). From a psychoanalytic perspective, in a pre-capitalist system, individuals are externally coerced and enslaved to become an object of the master's desire. In contrast, in a capitalist system, the master creates a framework of desire, leading the individual proletariats to consent to this capitalist-meritocratic system, essentially becoming voluntary participants in their own subjugation. Capitalism functions as an Other, generating a specific fantasy based on meritocratic doctrine by promising an improved quality of life, prosperity, fairness, justice, higher rate of salary, promotions, and social mobility for all proletariat individuals. However, this ideal of meritocracy is ultimately an illusion. It contributes to the deepening of structural inequality and suppresses the potential for social change that was anticipated by Marx, particularly the abolition of capitalism itself. The proletariat eventually recognizes this illusion, but they ironically and collectively choose to maintain the enjoyment that capitalism and the ideology of meritocracy provide.

To give an example, the tech industry frequently asserts that it operates on meritocratic principles, and there is a reason to question its narrative (Castilla, 2025, p. 4). Although tech companies have pledged to enhance diversity, access to capital and a corporate privilege status remain a significant barrier for many proletariats, particularly for minorities and women. These proletariats may face long hours, low pay, and minimal benefits. Despite these betrayals, they still take it as an enjoyment. Ironically, they still have a sense of loyalty to their company, a passion to work for their company, and derive satisfaction from their work. Hence, saying that Sunday evening is the time when the proletariat feels dread is not sufficient. The truly alarming aspect is that some members of the proletariat seem to take masochistic form of self-enjoyment by satisfying and exploiting themselves at work from Monday morning to Friday afternoon. This option of self-suffering enjoyment can undermine the potential for Marxism to foster class consciousness among the proletariat. This combination of pleasure and pain highlights the complexities of proletariat's self-masochistic enjoyment within a capitalist system of desire, illustrating how proletariats cope with unmet expectations for fulfillment and well-being.

This situation epitomizes the masochistic self-enjoyment of the proletariat. From the psychoanalytic perspective of the proletariat, who has become disillusioned with this object of desire yet continues to consume and enjoy it, capitalism can be likened to a maternal body, and the proletariat are like children addicted to her breast. This analogy illustrates how capitalism elicits a complex mix of love and hate within the proletariat. Therefore, a critique of capitalism cannot simply focus on the structural inequalities associated with wealth accumulation and exploitation, which lead to the emergence of the proletariat's class consciousness. This useful but outdated approach overlooks the important aspect of the proletariat's masochistic self-enjoyment that the capitalist system cultivates, which can hinder the development of class consciousness. Theoretically, class consciousness remains significant for the revolutionary movement. But, even if the proletariat achieves class consciousness, it is possible that their masochistic self-enjoyment may ultimately lead them to live, work, and die for capitalism, resulting in class consciousness fading away. This is a challenge that traditional Marxism should not ignore, as they may be overly optimistic about the prospects for class consciousness.

Ultimately, one could argue that Marx is the one who identifies the symptoms of capitalism because he focuses on the proletariat as a living being – the free laborer who must sell their labor power and life, only to be reduced to raw materials, tools, and means of production, even vital resources for the capitalist (Marx, 2024, p. 63). However, this perspective is contentious. It is important to note that capitalism undoubtedly represents a theater of cruelty for the proletariat, as argued by Marx. But what is dismissed by Marx is that capitalism is at the same time the theater of masochistic enjoyment and that the proletariat's lack of desire and fantasy as a fulfillment of lack is psychoanalytically related to it. Psychoanalysis raises a contentious issue regarding this aspect of enjoyment of the proletariat. Similar to the lethal form of alienation argued in the previous chapter, capitalism persists not only through new production means and technology but also because the proletariat actively finds enjoyment in a self-commoditization and willingly embraces their role within it until a loathe form of alienation is suppressed by the proletariat themselves, leading to the continuity of capitalism.

Sadistic enjoyment

The second pathological existence of the proletariat is sadistic enjoyment. In this context, enjoyment manifests within the individual as they find pleasure in violating and transgressing social obligations, even infringing upon the rights of others. When the enjoyment derived from such transgressions goes unmitigated and profoundly unchecked, it can compel the individual to repeat these acts that are uncomfortable for others to witness. This action is the root of sadism. Lacan refers to this situation as "the paradox of *jouissance*" (Lacan, 2008e, p. 237). In contrast to Aristotle's concept of eudaimonia, which signifies a flourishing state that benefits all and goes beyond mere personal happiness, Lacan presents the paradox of enjoyment through what he terms a "dialectic of happiness" (Lacan, 2008e, p. 237). This Hegelian dialectic suggests that enjoyment is not derived from adhering to the Law – conceived as an inviolable authority – but from viewing the Law as a mystically obscene Other. By questioning and negating the perception of the Law's supreme authority and adopting a skeptical stance toward this Other, individuals engage in a process of demystification. They rebel against the Law, disrupt social norms, and challenge public perception to gain a sadistic form of enjoyment.

Lacan's thesis on sadistic enjoyment draws from his critical interpretation of Christianity, as well as his reinterpretation of Sade and Kant in the context of psychoanalysis. For many conservative advocates of Kantian thought, concepts like the Law – which represents the metaphysical existence of divine entity, moral duty, and universal principles – act as assurances of transcendental happiness. Lacan suggests that the Other, or the Law, strives to see its own transcendental image reflected in the depths of a subject's unconscious. However, when the Other attempts to project its transcendental image onto the subject's unconscious, it does not signify a direct equivalence between the subject and the Other. Instead, it represents the Other's own death as a signifier of nothingness (Lacan, 2008e, p. 237). Since the Other is assumed as a void and embodies impossibility, this leads to a different form of surplus that goes beyond mere transcendental happiness. This idea is linked to enjoyment, and Lacan's concept of enjoyment is closely associated with his psychoanalytic radicalization of Kantian imperative: Kant's objective is not to comply with the Law but to desire to transgress it.

Essentially, beyond the Aristotelian concept of collective flourishing, which includes a faith in a monotheistic God, a voice of enjoyment emerges that relates to the transgression of laws and hegemonic social norms. This is captured in the sentence: "I retreat from loving my neighbor as myself because there is something on the horizon there that is engaged in some form of intolerable cruelty. In that sense, to love one's neighbor may be the cruelest of choices" (Lacan, 2008e, p. 239). If the Law fails to sustain happiness, or if it becomes a dead signifier, a sadistic form of enjoyment will be tangible in opposition to that regulative Law. For the sake of sadistic form of enjoyment that transgresses governing social norms – which are established in the name of a moral imperative aimed at preventing enjoyment – "man's rebellion is involved here, the rebellion of *jedermann*, of everyman" (Lacan, 2008e, p. 239). Inasmuch as he aspires to derive enjoyment, the truth that man seeks enjoyment at the expense of transgressing Law remains true. The sadistic form of enjoyment manifests a resistance to the commandment, "'Thou shalt love thy neighbor as thyself' and the resistance that is exercised to prevent access to *jouissance* are one and the same thing" (Lacan, 2008e, p. 239).

From this point, Lacan evokes the image of Sade by linking the Sadean experience to sadistic enjoyment. Lacan presents Sade as "the man of pleasure" (Lacan, 2008e, p. 245), the very same Sade who embodies a sadist enjoyment. The most paradoxical viewpoint is that Sadean enjoyment represents Kant's hidden desire. Kant's true desire is that he is a Sadean, but Sade is not Kantian. Lacan notes that "the great joy with which he recalls the emergence of this tradition historically is a clear sign of the point the master always reaches when he does not bow his head before the being of God" (Lacan, 2008e, p. 245). It is important to recognize that both the words "he" and "master" in this sentence refer to Sade. In other words, the sadistic form of enjoyment differs from the Christian law, which affirmatively commands individuals to love one another and to refrain from claiming rights over others' bodies. In a Sadean experience, the resistance to this law suggests a belief that "I have the right to enjoy your body" (Lacan, 2006b, p. 648). This essentializes a sadistic form of enjoyment, where enjoyment obtained from breaking another person's body into pieces is expressed – "my neighbor's body breaks into pieces" (Lacan, 2008e, 249): this symbolizes a mutual desire of Kant and Sade. Enjoyment here is closely tied to the sadistic subject and is significantly associated with the psychoanalytic concept of the "part object".

In a perspective that contrasts with Lacanian theories, particularly Melanie Klein's object relations theory. The Kleinian concept of the part object is viewed as the fetish object of love, tenderness, and hate that such ambiguity in the object paradoxically gives enjoyment to the subject (Mitchell and Black, 2016, p. 99). From a Kleinian viewpoint, the part object represents an imaginary entity that fosters personality, negating a sin of splitting, culminating in a cohesive communal bond (Klein, 1975, pp. 94–121). This includes forming communal relationships such as family and sexuality, and these connections are often maintained and solidified by a shared utopian fantasy that involves opposing enemies. Ultimately, such utopian fantasy is noted as a defensive mechanism developed by the psyche to fend off deepening conflicts, such as "the deep terrors of annihilation" (paranoid anxiety) and "utter abandonment" (depressive anxiety) within the communal relationships (Mitchell and Black, 2016, pp. 87–88). However, Lacan reinterprets this idea, moving away from Klein's view of the part object that is coalesced with a communal fostering among the subjects. Rather, he posits that the part object is inevitably linked to the enjoyment associated with Sadean experiences, which are rooted in the radical subject. This culminates in a rejection of any utopian fantasy promoted by Klein. Also, unlike Kant, who emphasizes moral imperatives, Lacan illustrates through Sade that the part object can bring satisfaction, which involves the subject offering a part of his or her body as a source of pleasure, even if it is painful, to the Other's existence. But in return, the Other's existence provides similar satisfaction to the subject, promising the sadistic form of enjoyment to the subject: the Other offers itself as the instrument of enjoyment for the subject. While the existence of the Other is seen as creating an alienating effect for the subject, the sadistic subject is one who inflicts pain upon the Other to ultimately deny the Other's existence (Lacan, 2006b, pp. 654–656). In contrast to Christian doctrines that promote love and tenderness among individuals, and against Aristotle's idea of teleological eudaimonia, this Sadean expression highlights the subject's enjoyment derived from others' bodies, as well as the subject's own body being sacrificed to provide enjoyment to others. The sadistic enjoyment derived from social transgression is evident in Sade's belief in the illusion of the Other as an unyielding presence. This enjoyment arises when the subject perceives the Other, such as the Law, as a potential victim, as a target for the transgressing act to invest in it (Lacan, 2008e, p. 249). For example, a serial killer obtains enjoyment by violating the laws set by the government and police. To maintain this form of enjoyment without any sense of lack, a sadistic individual, like a serial killer, feels compelled to repeatedly breach the Law: a metaphysical existence of the moral ruling paradigm. In this sense, enjoyment is linked to the subject, while the Other is not only non-intrusive but also infinitely vulnerable to violation.

Lacan's sadistic form of enjoyment is also explored in "A Theoretical Introduction to the Functions of Psychoanalysis in Criminology". He examines this idea by analyzing the relationship between the id, criminal behavior, and a lack of satisfaction. A sadistic individual is not categorized as merely a madman or an irrational person. Instead, a sadistic subject experiences an ineffable enjoyment that is dominated by the id without their conscious awareness. This is reflected in Lacan's statement that "the subject's 'tendencies' do not fail, moreover, to manifest slippage in relation to their level of satisfaction" (Lacan, 2006a, p. 122). It is important to recognize that enjoyment has a dangerous psychological aspect, particularly for individuals who actively choose to reject civic norms meant to regulate and control excessive levels of satisfaction. Therefore, enjoyment should not be viewed as a concept that Lacan endorses without critical examination. Rather, enjoyment ought to be understood as an uncanny trait in humanity. Lacan's notion of enjoyment, which stands in opposition to the conservative realization of Kantian moral imperative, offers an alternative hypothesis regarding civilization and its discontent. This perspective moves beyond Freud's original hypothesis, which primarily focuses on the displeasure associated with sexual restrictions. Lacan emphasizes the inherent psychological dangers within humanity, particularly among those who embody the signs of societal discord, such as madmen, serial killers, warmongers, and jingoists.

It is important to note that the proletariat is not exempt from this type of sadistic self-enjoyment. Considering the form of enjoyment discussed by Lacan reveals a discrepancy between his ideas and those of Marx. Lacan's concept of enjoyment, viewed as a form of social transgression, prompts a reconsideration of how this enjoyment characterizes the Marxist proletariat – a perspective that Marx seems to overlook. It is the enjoyment that arises from the exploitation among the proletariat, not in a classical sense that represents the capitalist's exploitation of the proletariat. As Lacan argues, "We would better to learn from it the lesson contained in a fine little tale told about the exploitation of one man by another, which is the definition of capitalism" (Lacan, 2006b, p. 656). In other words, the self-enjoyment of the proletariat, understood through Lacan's lens, presents the proletariat as a sadistic subject – one that has undergone Sadean experiences fundamental to its existence within the proletariat. If the proletariat is viewed as a sadistic subject or a person seeking pleasure, a troubling outcome is that they may exploit the bodies of other proletariats for their own enjoyment. This enjoyment would lead to a depoliticized evasion of the collective struggle against capitalism. Consequently, capitalism would continue, appearing as though it had never been overthrown, ultimately resulting in disappointment for Marx.

Instead of advocating for revolution and emancipatory politics, or expressing collective anger against the capitalist system, psychoanalysis cautions that the proletariat may find satisfaction in exploiting other members of the proletariat as a means to attain enjoyment, replacing the need for revolutionary politics. In his article "On the Jewish Question", Marx asserts that "political emancipation is also the dissolution of the old society, on which rests the state that is estranged from the people – the sovereign power" (Marx, 2007, p. 47). Optimistically, he further explains that political emancipation, viewed through the lens of a united proletariat acting as a rational agency, is characterized as "the political revolution that toppled this sovereign power and elevated state matters to the status of concerns of the people, thereby transforming the political state into a universal concern" (Marx, 2007, p. 48). However, from a psychoanalytic reading of Marx's idea, Marx's call for proletariat solidarity is met with skepticism. It is undermined by the proletariat's sadistic self-enjoyment. This raises concerns about Marx's emphasis on the proletariat as a political agency, highlighting the problematic nature of his perspective, and this prompts a traditional Marxism's re-evaluation of Marxist revolutionary theories centered on the proletariat, which often omits a psychoanalytic viewpoint.

One example of the dynamics among members of the proletariat experiencing a sadistic enjoyment and using each other's bodies as part objects for enjoyment can be seen in office politics. In today's competitive work environment, many of them experience stress, jealousy, mental health issues, and envy due to unequal treatment. Instead of confronting and affronting the capitalist system, these individuals often choose to depoliticize their situations. In their pursuit of recognition, career advancement, and higher status, they may resort to bullying one another, harassing, blaming their bosses, damaging their colleagues' reputations, and engaging in other harmful behaviors. This treatment reduces each other to mere part objects, with instances of bullying occurring both in person and online in order to obtain sadistic enjoyment (Neuman and Baron, 2011, p. 215). Ultimately, rather than addressing the capitalist system as the root cause, some proletariats derive a sadistic form of enjoyment from the emotional and psychological harm inflicted on their colleagues, leaving capitalism unscathed.

As the proletariat experiences sadistic enjoyment, it can lead to widespread depoliticization among them. Office politics should be condemned because it represents a distorted form of politics. This situation is problematic because the workplace politics easily leads to a violation of the moral principle – the Law of the Other – that everyone is supposed to show tenderness, care, and "love our neighbor (such as our colleagues) as ourselves". Additionally, office politics prompts the proletariat to seek organizational reform, striving for greater equality and improved relationships between bosses and subordinates in the workplace as a means of achieving freedom and liberation. When abusive behavior is tolerated as a source of enjoyment among proletariats in the modern spaces called offices and workplaces, it poses a significant challenge for Marxist politics. These scenarios demonstrate that some members of the proletariat may believe they have the right to derive satisfaction from the suffering of their fellow proletariat members, until a solidarity among global proletariat is at risk to be Marxist's Kantian idealization. Ironically, a new fantasy that will replace the neoliberal fantasy is the belief that an alternative mode of production, including a classless society, will provide all proletariats with perpetual peace.

Narcissistic enjoyment

The third pathological existence of the proletariat is narcissistic enjoyment. Such enjoyment arises from the subject's inclination toward narcissism. Narcissism is defined as a preoccupation with extreme self-centeredness, where the individual overvalues themselves and lacks empathy for the suffering of others. Narcissism is deeply rooted in the subject's anxiety about a potential lack of admiration and respect from others. This unconscious sense of inadequacy leads the narcissistic individual to demand excessive self-esteem from those around them. The narcissistic subject exists within the socio-symbolic realm of language. They recognize that language is essential to the development of their personality. According to Lacan, the narcissistic individual perceives the symbolic order as a vital source of enjoyment. Lacan states that "it is the symbolic order which is constitutive for the subject – by demonstrating in a story the major determination the subject receives from the itinerary of a signifier" (Lacan, 2006c, p. 7).

Narcissistic enjoyment is characterized by a strong addiction to the symbolic order, which fosters condescension and complacency in the grand persona of the narcissist. This type of individual demands to be an essential part of the field of the Other. A narcissistic form of enjoyment stems from the desire expressed by the Other, shaping their subjectivity. It is possible that the unconscious serves as a defense against recognizing this desire of the Other, separating from the ego (Lacan, 2006d, p. 355). But for the narcissistic enjoyment, it remains caught in a symptomatic unity between ego and unconscious, preventing the subject from realizing their authentic self. Instead of evolving a true identity, the narcissist clings to a false image, reliant on the desires of the Other. Consequently, speech becomes infused with this external desire, making it impossible for a narcissist to separate enjoyment from the influence of the Other, resulting in a mature form of narcissism that thrives within the symbolic order.

Narcissistic enjoyment stems from Freud's original thesis. Freud presents narcissism not merely as a form of sexual energy or libido but as a psychological drive that exists outside the reality that shapes the individual. This thesis is more nuanced than it initially appears. Freud suggests that narcissism arises from the subject's focus and emotional investment in "object-cathexes", which are the objects that engage the subject's psychological energies, including sexual instincts and desires transferred by the subjects to the libido objects (Freud, 2003, p. 5). When the subject successfully fulfills, possesses, and controls these objects of desire, they are gratified by this object of libido and ultimately enjoy a psychological state characterized by self-narcissism (Freud, 2003, p. 29). Lacan expands on this by considering the object-cathexes as the things the Other demands that the subject pursue, consume, and possess. For the subject, fulfilling desires regarding these objects leads to a state of symptomatic entropy. Unfortunately, the outcome of this cycle is ultimately dissatisfaction, yet the narcissistic subject continues to derive enjoyment from repeating it. They seek satisfaction from various object-cathexes available within the field of the Other. This cycle will persist indefinitely unless there is a complete cessation of enjoyment derived from the relationship between the narcissistic subject and the object-cathexes. Since the narcissistic subject thrives on this enjoyment within the realm of the Other, the cycle tends to resume, and any political negation of this loop is often disregarded.

At this point, another theoretical perspective regarding Marx's proletariat and Lacanian psychoanalysis can be explored. Marx does not adequately depict the proletariat as experiencing narcissistic enjoyment. This implies that the psychological realm of the proletariat is significantly shaped, if not overwhelmed, by a form of narcissistic enjoyment, which is a key characteristic of their self-satisfaction. Considering the proletariat as a narcissistic subject prevalent in workplaces prompts the idea that they are highly self-centered and demonstrate a lack of compassion for their fellow proletariats. In competitive environments, capitalism provides the narcissistic proletariat with various opportunities, such as social mobility through career promotions, professional development, and motivation for entrepreneurship by starting their own businesses. The intense focus on self-interest leads to diminished empathy for others. Therefore, it is reasonable to discuss the self-exploitation of the proletariat in pursuit of the benefits that capitalism offers. In consequence, the presence of narcissistic enjoyment in the narcissistic proletariat leads to the disintegration of a cohesive proletarian bloc, hindering any collective resistance against capitalist hegemony. Psychoanalysis highlights the proletariat's inclination toward narcissism – seeking social acceptance, fame, mobility, and recognition – often at the cost of the suffering and despair of their fellow proletariats.

Furthermore, it is important to examine the similarities and differences between the narcissistic proletariat and the lumpenproletariat (Marx, 2021, p. 38). A key difference lies in the lumpenproletariat's refusal to recognize themselves as part of the oppressed class. This group includes individuals such as the unemployed, homeless, and criminals, who are often excluded from capitalist production. In contrast, narcissistic proletariats are typically employed and registered workers in various workplaces. While the lumpenproletariat, including the poor and beggars, exists outside the capitalist system, the narcissistic proletariat is integrated into it. Unlike lumpenproletariat, they are aware of class consciousness and class antagonism. They know how they are exploited and treated as instruments within the capitalist framework, but they seek success within capitalism, often resorting to unethical means to achieve their goals. As they navigate their lives as money machines for mere sustenance, regulated by the demands of capitalism, it is difficult to expect them to exhibit collective empathy. Moreover, the narcissistic proletariat struggles to adhere to Susan Sontag's ethical imperative of "regarding the pain of others" (Sontag, 2003). They often perceive the suffering of fellow proletariats as a source of enjoyment in the capitalist environment, which further detaches them from a sense of shared political ideology, namely, an abolition of capitalism.

In his original framework, Marx defines the proletariat as a class of laborers who do not own means of production, such as machinery, technology, or advanced equipment. This idea is particularly highlighted in Marx's work "Machinery and Modern Industry", where he elaborates on this aspect.

> On a closer examination of the working machine proper, we find in it, as a general rule, though often, no doubt, under very altered forms, the apparatus and tools used by the handicraftsman or manufacturing workman; with this difference, that instead of being human implements, they are the implements of mechanism, or mechanical implements.
>
> (Marx, 2013, pp. 257–258)

The statement clearly defines the proletariat, including individuals such as "handicraftsmen or manufacturing workers", as those who utilize industrial tools – object-cathexes – provided by capitalists, the owners of such technology. The entire production process highlights the reality and power dynamics established by machinery, which can replace the labor force of the proletariat. Marx characterizes the proletariat as laborers who lack ownership of the means of production. He estimates that the proletariat will eventually be replaced by advancements in industrial machinery. In Marx's view,

> the machine, which is the starting-point of the industrial revolutions, supersedes the workman, who handles a single tool, by a mechanism operating with a number of similar tools, and set in motion by a single motive power, whatever the form of that power may be. Here, we have the machine, but only as an elementary factor of production by machiner.
>
> (Marx, 2013, p. 259)

Significantly, Žižek contrasts Marx's view of the proletariat by arguing that the contemporary proletariats, like Uber drivers, are paradoxically the "small capitalists" (Novara Media, 2025), who use the means of production for their own benefit and enjoy the freedom in capitalism. He suggests that the modern proletariat is a precarious worker who chooses between jobs rather than being alienated by capitalism. This indicates that the identity of the proletariat can perpetuate capitalism without significant ideological change, as they may willingly objectify and self-alienate themselves. This perspective diverges from traditional Marxist views. Following Žižek, it can be said that while technology serves as the means of production owned by the capitalist, it becomes something the proletariat becomes familiar with during the production process. Consequently, proletariat knows how to possess, acquire, and utilize the means of production. Owning the means of production may lead to a narcissistic enjoyment among some proletariats, particularly those who achieve social mobility by eventually becoming capitalists themselves. Now, as the narcissistic capitalist subjects, these former proletariats might choose to oppress or subdue other proletariats rather than empathize with them. Also, they often take pleasure in the commodities produced within the capitalist framework, resulting in a significant divide within the proletariat class. This situation aligns with Lacan's warning about the challenging relationship between individuals, such as the proletariat, and object-cathexes, such as the means of production. The latter may consist of technologies and gadgets that the proletariat might ultimately choose not to use these object-cathexes for political revolutionary purposes. Lacan's critique of Marx at this point is outstanding:

> You would be wrong to think that the relation of man to the object of his production as its fundamental level has been completely elucidated – even by Marx, who took things very far in this respect.
>
> (Lacan, 2008d, p. 279)

In capitalism, a narcissistic proletariat, who can advance to become a capitalist, often feels inadequate and insecure due to a culture of competition. This sense of lack drives the quest for new marketing strategies and innovative products. To sustain their narcissistic enjoyment from this deficiency, they delve deeper into the capitalist system, seeking survival and achievement from the capitalist red sea system, which can lead to the oppression of fellow proletariats. As a result, the hope for political solidarity among the proletariat may appear futile and overly optimistic, reflecting challenges within traditional Marxist theory.

The three psychoanalytic dimensions of enjoyment – masochistic, sadistic, and narcissistic – are interconnected in the individuality of the proletariat and play a significant role in sustaining capitalism. To clarify, masochistic enjoyment arises from pursuing objects that do not align with the proletariat's true desires; however, they may pretend to accept these objects as if they genuinely desire them. In contrast, sadistic enjoyment is exhibited through the depoliticized and harmful behaviors of the proletariat, such as workplace bullying, which can hinder authentic political action aimed at discovering alternatives to capitalism. Narcissistic enjoyment is evident among successful members of the proletariat who, in turn, become exploiters themselves. These three interconnected dimensions of proletariat's self-enjoyment illustrate how a single proletariat individual can embody multiple forms of enjoyment, highlighting a pathological existence that perpetuates capitalism. This does not mean that the proletariat lacks class consciousness. Rather, assuming they already possess class consciousness, these three forms of enjoyment often become objects of fetishism for the proletariat. Unlike the lumpenproletariat, they are aware of their class consciousness in relation to a structural class conflict lodged in capitalism, but they enjoy ignoring it. However, these three forms of self-enjoyment can become the fetishisms that ultimately undermine their class consciousness and weaken the revolutionary ideology of the proletariat – an aspect of psychoanalysis that Marx and traditional Marxism fail to address.

The revolutionary proletariat subject as Lacanian Woman

The not-whole

Marx argues that women are exploited as a means of production, emphasizing that capitalism systematically oppresses women's lives. Marx and Engels (2004) assert that communism will inspire "an openly legalized community of women" (p. 44), but he often faces illegitimate criticism from liberal feminists for their inadequate theoretical and conceptual approach regarding women's subjectivities (Weinbaum, 1978, pp. 34–46: Holmstrom, 1981, p. 194). Upon reflection, there are two key aspects overlooked by both Marx and liberal feminism. First, Marx fails to recognize how women's subjectivity – particularly the Lacanian concept of Woman and her enigmatic desires – could inspire a reimagining of the proletariat as a radically sacred subject. Second, liberal feminism also neglects to consider the connection between the proletariat and women's desires, which are intertwined with the notion of divine enjoyment. This understanding could allow for the proletariat's subjectivity to be deontologized and depathologized from the three modes of self-enjoyment – masochism, sadism, and narcissism – discussed in the previous section.

This section will depart from the pathological existence of the proletariat's self-enjoyment by introducing a more radicalized version of the subjectivity of the proletariat in relation to the three logics of the Lacanian woman, derived from Lacan's teachings. It is important to note that all three logics of the Lacanian woman – the not whole, the divine enjoyment, and Antigone – are situated beyond gender difference, as these theoretical perspectives can also be applied to male proletariats. The objective is to demonstrate how the concept of the Lacanian woman is epistemologically linked to Marx's politics of proletariat emancipation, as well as informing Marx's limitations.

The first concept of Lacanian psychoanalysis regarding the proletariat subject that Marx is blinded to is the idea that proletariats are Lacanian woman characterized as "not whole". This notion might be unsettling for some Marxist-Feminist scholars, especially in light of Lacan's statements about women, such as "woman does not exist" (Lacan, 1999c, p. 7). Lacan's portrayal of women is more radical and can significantly contribute to the subject of liberation, more than they may realize, though Lacan's representation of women also has deficiencies and limitations. When considering political revolution, proletariat subjects should not omit Lacan's idea of the "not-whole". This concept suggests that women cannot be reduced to or viewed as mere objects of phallic desire or enjoyment over their bodies (Lacan, 1999c, p. 7).

In the diagram (see Figure 5.1), it is evident that the woman, depicted as being associated with phallic enjoyment – the Other (A) – is essentially a barred woman, as shown in the lower right column (Lacan, 1999a, p. 78). A woman in relation to phallic enjoyment is the barred subject, represented as \$, indicated in the lower left column. However, Lacan recognizes that the woman possesses a remainder; she is the *objet a* (*a*), or a signifier that forms a non-relationship within every discourse, serving as an externality, even as an excess, to the impotent male gaze (barred A). In relation to male phallic enjoyment, the woman, as a lacking or incomplete entity, is designated as the *objet a* (see Figure 5.1). This designation creates a mystique around the image of woman that has the potential to disrupt the phallic enjoyment that men have claimed. Mapping an image of woman with the phallic enjoyment is a lack of totality, since woman is the "signifier that has no signified" (Lacan, 1999a, p. 81), which Lacan designates the symbol of empty set, Ø, as having an excessive yet mystical characteristic that forms a disparity constituted in the phallic enjoyment. Proletariat subjects, insofar as the emancipatory politics is concerned, should form and renew their ground of being identical to Lacan's woman as a not-whole, creating confusion and disturbance to the phallic field of capitalism.

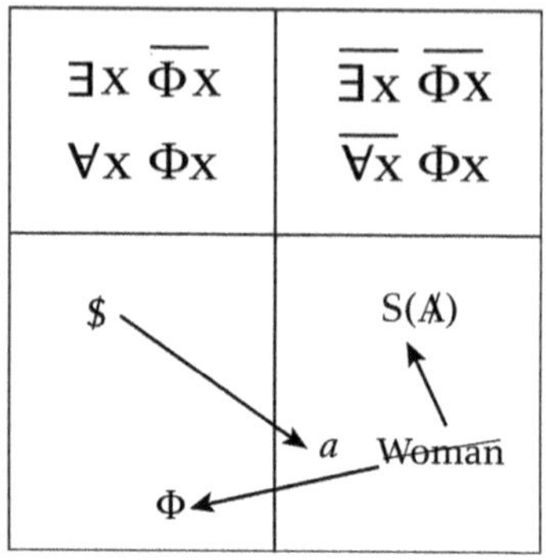

Figure 5.1 Lacan's logic of sexuation.

Source: Figure adapted from Lacan, J. (1999). *The Seminar of Jacques Lacan Book XX: On Feminine Sexuality*. Edited by Jacques-Alain Miller. Translated by Bruce Fink. London and New York: W.W. Norton Company. p. 78.

Regardless of differences in gender and sexuality, a proletariat subject should embrace Lacan's concept of the woman as not-whole. This theoretical stance provides an emotional counterargument and simultaneously a rejection of the proletariat's self-enjoyment. The statement "woman does not exist" was never meant by Lacan to diminish the value of women. Instead, Lacan suggests that a woman, as a "being-not-whole", experiences a type of contingent enjoyment that differs from what the phallic function designates as consistent enjoyment (Lacan, 1999b, p. 73). As this mystical form of enjoyment indicates, the idea of a universal essence of woman does not hold up within the realm of phallic enjoyment (Lacan, 1999b, pp. 72–73). Marx's concept of the proletariat should follow this possible imagination. When discussing proletariat's enjoyment as a designation of Ø, it becomes clear that there is no universal essence of the proletariat's desire within the context of capitalism, nor within the three modes of proletariat self-enjoyment that sustain capitalism: masochism, sadism, and narcissism.

Divine enjoyment

A second aspect of the Lacanian notion of woman relates to Lacan's unconventional view of Catholicism. This is also vital for the reinterpretation of Marx's conception of the proletariat. Lacan's discussion of God presents God as an embodiment of divine enjoyment, as akin to a woman's undefined and excessive enjoyment. This theological perspective suggests a connection between the subject of the proletariat and Marxist theoretical discussions. In Seminar XX, Lacan refers to God's enjoyment or divine enjoyment as the "Supreme Being's *jouissance*, that is, God's" (Lacan, 1999b, p. 70). Lacan poses an intriguing psychoanalytic question: does God Himself know that He is revered by mortals as the Supreme Being? It seems that Lacan implies that the Biblical representation of God as the Supreme Being, correlated with the Trinity – God, the Son, and the Spirit – might obscure a true understanding of God's enjoyment – a divine or Supreme Being's enjoyment – which is related to the question of how God exactly perceives Himself. Lacan further explores the concept of God's enjoyment in *The Triumph of Religion* (2013), where his critical stance toward God reflects a degree of skepticism about God being presupposed as the Name-of-the-Father, the creator of the world who possesses a divine love granted to all humanity.

Lacan focuses on the Christian monotheistic God rather than other religions or polytheistic deities. In Lacan's framework, the Christian God is ontologically challenged and dialectically opposed, which allows for a transformation from a fatherly image of gentle kindness to an antithetical representation that negates its original form. Since divine enjoyment is naturally contingent, humans perceive this supreme enjoyment as excessive, mutually incomprehensible, and unsurpassable. Thus, divine enjoyment is considered the Real, referring to an impossible element that cannot be symbolized in definitive knowledge within public consciousness. At this juncture, Lacan also introduces the concept of consistent enjoyment – a symbolization of enjoyment through a signifier that is viable and constant – contrasting it with contingent enjoyment, which represents the Real indicative of divine enjoyment. As a result, the God depicted in the Bible serves as an object of desire for believers within a symbolic framework. This representation of God as the Father of Love in the Trinity emphasizes a consistent sense of enjoyment, embodying the fantasy of a generous, protective masculine Father watching over His mortal sons. In contrast, God's enjoyment is connected to the concept of the Real, which represents enjoyment as an uncanny "Thing" that transcends conventional biblical interpretation (Lacan, 2013, p. 50). For Lacan, this Real aspect of divine enjoyment – characterized by its excessive and unsignified nature – is linked to what Lacan terms the "Thing", which signifies the horror of such divine enjoyment that features woman's enjoyment. In Lacan's own words, "Thanks to which, naturally, you are going to be convinced that I believe in God. I believe in the *jouissance* of woman insofar as it is extra (*en plus*)" (Lacan, 1999b, pp. 76–77, italics original). Arguably, the only concept of God that seems fitting for this time of political turmoil is that of an all-encompassing, indifferent God (Žižek, 2025, p. 38), which transcends the fantasy construction found in biblical representations. This reflects the apathy entity, whose divine enjoyment tears apart the fantasy construction of God in the biblical representation.

Divine enjoyment is not merely a celestial form of enjoyment; rather, it is an experience that is deeply connected to the lives of mortal humans. Psychoanalysis suggests that a genuine existence of God does not hinge on the authority of God as presented biblically as a Love of the Father. Instead, it revolves around daring to believe in a divine enjoyment, which is understood as both ontologically and contingently excessive. Since this God's enjoyment designates a particular form of enjoyment experienced by women, this concept of divine enjoyment opens a space for a post-secular understanding of God – one that minimally diverges from secularism, evangelism, and atheism. A post-secular God is not envisioned as a Supreme Being as a transcendental entity, nor a divine entity out-of-joint dissociated from the lives of the mortal beings but rather as a deity-man hybridization characterized by excessive, unsignified, and contingent enjoyment, akin to the enjoyment of woman. This idea aligns with Lacan's assertion, "I believe in God" and "I believe in the *jouissance* of woman insofar as it is extra", as mentioned earlier. This Lacanian thought about God converges with Benedict Spinoza's view of God not as a transcendent entity but as an active presence that connects with mortal beings. Spinoza's God is an immanent Being that enables humans to develop rational potential and acquire knowledge, which can then be used to create social bonds and connections with one another. Fundamentally, this post-secularized notion of God, or God embodied in human mortals, is ontologically the subject who has experienced excessive and contingent enjoyment, particularly in relation to women. This understanding is why Lacan reinterprets Fyodor Dostoevsky's famous quote, "If there is no God, everything is permitted", to mean, "If there is a God, then anything is permitted" (Žižek, 2024). This means dangerously that for those who refer to God directly, believing themselves to be instruments of His will, nothing is forbidden. Dostoevsky's view of God is rooted in a tradition of evangelism, reflecting human anxiety about sin and the punishment that comes from God. In contrast, similar to Spinoza's God, Lacan's God is perceived as an embodiment within humanity that can justify any human actions and experience divine enjoyment.

In contrast to Marx's atheism, it is suggested that the proletariat could revive and embody a post-secularized concept of God influenced by Lacan and Spinoza. For the proletariat to serve as a revolutionary radical subject, contemporary Marxist thought on political emancipation requires this reimagined idea of God. It is essential for the proletariat to adopt a notion of post-metaphysical God's enjoyment – a divine enjoyment – that aligns with a subjectivity conducive to political revolution. It is also essential for the proletariat to embrace the concept of women's enjoyment in the formation of their radical subjects. Historically, it is Marx's atheism and the hypothesis of women being oppressed by capitalism that fuel proletariat revolutions. But in the present, it is a post-secularized God embodied by the proletariat as akin to a figure of Lacanian woman that can inspire emancipatory politics, making the Marxist politics of emancipation seem to be the irreligiously feminine sacred – a divine enjoyment linked to a women's enjoyment that forms the proletariat's radical subjects. A key aspect of women's contingent enjoyment is its ability to disrupt the current reality of capitalism, which encompasses both the three modes of self-enjoyment of the proletariat, as noted earlier, and the phallic enjoyment often associated with capitalism. Thus, within this framework of divine enjoyment – the dialectic of proletariat's self-enjoyment – the proletariat increasingly needs this post-metaphysical concept of God, even though such a political interpretation of God embraced by the proletariat subject is different from Marx's atheism.

Antigone

A third logic on the Lacanian concept of woman that enables a reinterpretation of Marxism's proletariat subject is Lacan's interpretation of *Antigone*, a play by the ancient Greek tragedian Sophocles. In the storyline, Antigone is the daughter of Oedipus and his incestuous wife, Jocasta. The name Antigone itself means *one who is of the opposite opinion*. The name Antigone symbolizes the Lacanian woman as incomplete, creating a void in the realm of phallic enjoyment: precisely, Antigone is the Lacanian Real. Arguably, Lacan's interpretation of Antigone represents the Law of non-Christian God, whose divine enjoyment embodied in female body is contingent and mystical, capable of challenging male dominance, especially in her defiance of Creon, the male ruler of Thebes and Jocasta's brother. In adhering to God's demands, Antigone values familial ties over allegiance to Creon's political authority. Sophocles portrays her determination to bury her brother Polyneices, which ultimately leads to her tragic death and instigates a series of unfortunate events that cause suffering for Creon, his family, and result in a collapse of his autocratic regime.

Antigone represents a form of divine enjoyment that is not associated with traditional biblical values. Her death signifies not only a personal tragedy but also a challenge to Creon's political authority, symbolizing a disruption connected to phallic enjoyment. Lacan notes, "She lives in the house of Creon; she is subject to his law; and that is something that she cannot bear" (Lacan, 2008b, p. 323). Through the character of Antigone, a Lacanian woman displays an active subject rather than a passive, conservative figure. With her embodiment of the non-Christian God, she actively seeks to overturn the existing political order. This interpretation of the Lacanian woman contrasts sharply with the conception of women found in contemporary woke culture, including feminist wokeism, which often seeks equality within the current structure of male-dominant capitalism instead of striving to dismantle its oppressive elements. Antigone embodies a radicalized subjectivity as a Lacanian woman; she dares to confront the boundary between life and death, unlike some feminists who might feel deterred from taking such bold actions. This is why the enjoyment experienced by a Lacanian woman is considered mystical and transcends the limitations of phallic enjoyment. This dimension of thought is significant but is often overlooked by Marx's insights, especially when the figure of Antigone, as the embodiment of divine enjoyment, is suggested as the proletariat subject.

Antigone is destined for divine enjoyment through what seems like a divine decision. In Lacan's framework, divine enjoyment – associated with God as a natural presence or natural immanence in human lives – emerges within a symbolic order but is later stripped of its illusory symbolic meaning. A figure like Antigone occupies a precarious position between two forms of death. The first form is biological death, an inevitable physical end that everyone must face. The second form refers to divine death, which is linked to a divine decision or Fate. In this second form, she is meant to sacrifice her life against the city's oppressive regime that symbolizes Antigone's commitment to divine mission. Antigone's sacrificial existence embodies a contingent divine enjoyment. By upholding divine law and resisting the oppressive, phallic-autocratic symbolic order represented by Creon, she ultimately faces her sacrificial death. This fate, determined by God's mystical enjoyment from the beginning, encapsulates the essence of divine enjoyment.

All the aforementioned theoretical discussions could be submitted to Marx and traditional Marxism for reconsideration regarding an Antigonean subject of the proletariat capable of enacting a Lacanian woman's divine enjoyment. It appears that Marx and Marxist scholars in Anglo-Saxon academia are often preoccupied with the figure of Daniel Defoe's Robinson Crusoe, identifying him as the emerging capitalist individual. Crusoe embodies problematic traits, such as being a slave trader and a racist who sells opium in Bengal, while also supporting wars against Muslims worldwide. The paradox here is that the more Marxists engage with Crusoe, the more they inadvertently act as spokespersons for capitalism, and this unintentional apology for capitalism is the embarrassing situation for the Marxists. Continuing to discuss Crusoe may be intended as a critique of capitalism, but it does not result in the abolition of capitalism itself. Merely talking about Crusoe does not foster the development of a radical subject, especially regarding women as embodiments of divine enjoyment within the context of emancipatory politics. As a result, this embarrassing situation does not present a viable path out of capitalism. In contrast, by dismantling existing orders – like Creon's order and, indeed, capitalism in our current reality – one can explore a radical form of politico-psychoanalytic life such as Antigone. Antigone represents a woman subject stripped of the symbolic order, embodying a signifier of life that is, in itself, unsignified. Through Antigone, there is a particularity of life that Lacan terms *Ate*, which he defines as a life that refuses to be constrained by the limits of being human, happiness, and desire confined by the reality principle. Instead of the image of Crusoe, in which capitalism becomes more viable as long as this image is discussed, it is the image of Antigone that inevitably stretches "beyond the limits of human" (Lacan, 2008b, p. 324), transcending the boundaries associated with capitalism's reality principle.

Instead of Crusoe, Antigone serves as a more suitable figure for the formation of the proletariat subject. This means that the proletariat subject, which Marx envisioned as a political force for emancipation, should be represented not by Crusoe but by the unique aspects of Antigone's life. These aspects transcend the entire system of signifiers and moralities that are part of the reality principle. This shift can contribute to a radical act aimed at overthrowing capitalism. Antigone embodies the Real that resists all modes of symbolization associated with the reality of capitalism. When a subject engages in a radical act that exceeds the limits of *Ate*, this goes beyond mere self-immolation or the death drive. It contributes to a certain type of ethics that coordinates with the Lacanian concept of the subject, who "acts in conformity with one's desire" (Lacan, 2008f, p. 382), rather than act in conformity with social expectations. This action also rejects the hypocritical "demand for happiness" (Lacan, 2008c, p. 361), which defines happiness as the fulfillment of desires only within the constraints of capitalism's reality principle. Again, Antigone serves as a symbol of women's liberation, embodying her ethics through actions that correspond with her desires. This portrayal of Antigone, representing a state of enjoyment that transcends human limitations and connects to the existing reality, can also be interpreted as a potential representation of the proletariat subject. This subject, whose misguided actions may lead to ethical good, resonated with Lacan's perspective in the following:

> It is because man mistakes evil for the good, because something beyond the limits of *Ate* has become Antigone's good, namely a good that is different from everyone's else.
>
> (Lacan, 2008a, p. 333; italics originals)

It is psychoanalytically assumed that enjoyment has the characteristics of a Mobius Strip. The subject of the proletariat may embody this form of Antigonean divine enjoyment. However, this divine enjoyment can realistically be undermined and must be retracted, not due to external stimuli but due to internal factors. One could argue that this Antigonean divine enjoyment is unstable. It may regress and become agonized because of the influence of the three modes of self-enjoyment that interfere with it. In addition, Marx's Christian atheistic standpoint does not mean to deny Christianity as such but to enable Christian to be a true Christian. According to Marx, the true Christian is the Christian who has a socialist element: the true function of Christianity is to wholly oppose private property, the mode of capitalist production, marriage, and state authority (Marx and Engels, 2004, p. 51). Marx and Engels (2004) assert that "Christian Socialism is but the holy water with which the priest consecrates the heart-burnings of the aristocrat" (p. 51). It is the proletariat as a revolutionary agent as promoting Christian Socialism "to pave the way for the new social Gospel" (Marx and Engels, 2004, p. 60): it seems that God imagined in this line of thought is God external to capitalism's fidelity to Him but God as a proponent of communism, where he is treated equal to Men, or even no more needs to exist. Hence, the communist world is a world that welcomes religion, or it is possible for a new mode of religion that promotes genuine equity to have room in the communist world.

In contrast to Marx's obsession with Christian Socialism, viewing the proletariat as an embodiment of Lacanian Antigonean divine enjoyment reveals that proletariat as a non-biblical God in themselves is not the same God as imagined in Marx's viewpoint on Christian Socialism. Through Antigonean divine enjoyment, this is why the proletariat's revolution and the communist imaginary do not promote a new egalitarian form of Christian Socialism. Unlike Marx, who imagines God separated from Men, it is the revolutionary proletariats who believe that all Men have God's enjoyment in themselves, and this inspires a passion for revolution. But it is this deity-human hybridization that is fragile and untenable and at risk of facing death like Antigone. Moreover, the "new social Gospel" remains Marx's *objet petit a*, in this sense, referring to an unattainable object that serves as the cause of desire of the subject. In addition, the "new social Gospel" also functions as a Marxist fantasy, since Marx was likely to be dismissed by the Real in the communist world that resisted his symbolization of communism. From a Lacanian perspective, the dialectic of enjoyment is internal to the proletariat, positioning them to stand at the threshold between capitalism and social change.

Rethinking Marx's concept of the proletariat does not involve merely reiterating it through a standard theory that Marx himself presupposes. As Žižek suggests regarding the true nature of the self,

> there is a human subject only within language, within a symbolic universe. Yet at the same time, we are never at home in language. There is always a gap; you say something, but you fail exactly to say what you want to say and so on. (The Institute of Art and Ideas, 2025)

This suggests that one can reinterpret and move beyond the assumptions and language presented by Marx – essentially, a Marxism's symbolic universe – by recognizing how Marx's inability to fully articulate the concept of the proletariat allows one to understand it deeper, to grasp its human subjectivity. In this context, the subjectivity of Marx's proletariat can find its true expression – its possible true home – only when it diverges from Marx's own linguistic framework.

Rethinking divine violence

To engage in political revolution, it is essential for the proletariat to rethink the thesis of divine violence as suggested by Slavoj Žižek in his book *Violence* (2008). Žižek (2008) argues that divine violence is distinct from other forms of violence, such as physical violence, systemic violence, and fanaticism, as it has a politically ideological nature that aims to dismantle the existing law (p. 178). In post-politics, political matters are left to the sovereign state; in post-ideology, violence by individuals often leads to self-immolation without challenging the regime. While other forms sustain the status quo in a post-political and post-ideological context, a form of divine violence aims for substantial change that points toward the mass unleashing of a repressed resentment (Žižek, 2008,

p. 188). Žižek's unique insight into divine violence advocates for a global approach to tackle pressing challenges such as environmental degradation, resource depletion, pandemics, and warfare. He emphasizes the urgent need for cooperation in what could be described as the world in the morning after. He rejects the ultra-Left's revival of Leninism as a viable solution to political deadlocks and critiques the pseudo-populist Left's focus on identity politics – specifically around national, gender, and racial differences – arguing that this focus serves as an obstacle to achieving genuine global cooperation.

Divine violence is a philosophical reflection rooted in Žižek's Lacanian-Hegelian Marxist framework. First, from a Lacanian framework, Žižek's divine violence is the Lacanian Real that resists the existing order of capitalism, neoliberal ideology, and postmodern politics. Second, from a Hegelian framework, Žižek's divine violence is characterized as a speculative subject, which Hegel describes as the "negation of negation" (Žižek, 2000, p. 70). This notion reflects a void of the impossible subject that is not assimilated into public consciousness. It nonetheless advocates a new form of the subject as a negativity who can menace the current symbolic order (Žižek, 2000, p. 72). According to Hegel's "negation of negation", divine violence emphasizes a thesis that provocatively contrasts with other forms of violence. Unlike physical violence, fanaticism, fascism, and systemic violence – each of which negates the previous one without effecting genuine historical change – divine violence seeks a radical transformation. Lastly, from a Marxist framework, Žižek's divine violence becomes a possibility for the politics of the proletariat and represents a collective revolutionary act capable of disrupting the systemic violence inherent in the cyclical nature of capitalism.

A new consideration of divine violence, or the proletariat subject experiencing divine enjoyment, is an aspect that Marx leaves unaddressed. Unlike other forms of violence that struggle to bring about social change, Žižek (2008) argues that divine violence is essential for realizing the aspirations of the traditional Left – "a positively existing historical phenomena" (p. 197) – that sustains the moderately conservative communist of his current standpoint. In Walter Benjamin's original thesis, divine violence embodies a celestial force of transcendence capable of disrupting human-made laws. Žižek seems to urge one to reinterpret this concept within a post-secular context, emphasizing the sovereignty of the people and the courage required to take destructive action against the immanent existing order. Consequently, divine violence is revamped as a thesis compatible with proletariat politics, serving as an antithesis to current wokeism and the Laclauian Left populism.

Rethinking the concept of divine violence through Žižek's framework from a Lacanian perspective reveals extensively the connections between the feminine logic of not-whole, divinity, and women's enjoyment embodied by the proletariat. It is important to understand divine violence not as an end in itself but as a political means for the proletariat to challenge the status quo. This form of violence is characterized by the Lacanian idea of woman's desire as incomplete, which poses a threat to the established order, particularly when other forms of violence and the Laclauian political ideology of pluralistic agonisms prove ineffective in dismantling oppressive socio-political structures. Divine violence is closely linked to the ethical principles embodied by Antigone. She represents divine enjoyment and exemplifies a radical act that transcends conventional limits, known as *Ate*, as noted earlier. Furthermore, rethinking divine violence necessitates recognizing the divine enjoyment of the proletariat, a synthesis of both God and mortal humanity within one's body and spirit. It is the Man who perceives himself as God that allows for God to exist as a pure immanence – a Being-in-the-world – which opens possibilities for social transformation.

Capitalism flourishes not only through imperialism and the military-industrial complex but also through a collective belief in theology, particularly Christianity. In other words, both Protestantism and Catholicism play an important role in the growth of capitalism rather than its decline: it is both Protestantism and Catholicism that underpin capitalism. The famous one is Max Weber's analysis of Protestant ethics, which highlights how virtues such as diligence and individualism promoted by Puritan ascetism, favored by God, contribute to the persistence of capitalism (Weber, 2001, p. 123). For Lacan, he views Catholicism as a factor that supports capitalist discourse, as illustrated by his discussion of Pascal's wager. This wager reflects the masochistic enjoyment of the proletariat, framed as an act of free will, where proletariats commoditize themselves as surplus-value within the capitalist system. The proletariat seeks to be useful to capitalists and ultimately renounces this enjoyment, convincing themselves that their actions, which favor the capitalist system, align with God's will. Consequently, they become increasingly involved in generating surplus-value for capitalism, thereby sustaining their masochistic enjoyment. This cycle perpetuates the enjoyment derived from the capitalist market, rooted in the proletariat's wager that God exists. (Lacan, 2024a, pp. 9–10).

Pascal's Wager suggests that if God exists and an individual chooses to believe, they stand to gain eternal happiness, which can be viewed psychoanalytically as a fantasy of the afterlife. On the other hand, if they choose not to believe, they risk facing eternal damnation. However, if God does not exist, believers do not lose anything of significant value. Therefore, it is more rational to embrace belief in God, as the potential benefits of belief outweigh the risks of disbelief, even in the absence of definitive proof of His existence. In this context, the rational proletariat is likely to reject Marx's atheism and choose not to abolish capitalism. The most significant benefit they anticipate is to choose to believe in God. By choosing to reject Marx's atheism, they may tolerate the oppressive regime of capitalism in the hopes of gaining eternal happiness – the fantasy of the afterlife – until death. Conversely, another option, if the proletariat decides not to believe in God, they may choose to fight against capitalism and work toward establishing a communist world where belief in God is absent. Here, they are likely to face two possible consequences in the communist world: first, if God exists, they will confront eternal damnation. Second, if God does not exist, they will lose nothing of significant value. Instead, it is divine violence that seeks to abolish capitalism, which can be beneficial for the politics of the proletariat within the framework of post-secular politics. Beyond Marx's imagination, who largely neglects the role of God embodied in the proletariat, it is the substantial image of unbiblical God embraced by the Antigonean proletariat mortals that has become increasingly relevant for contemporary proletariat politics.

Enjoyment as a political factor: a philosophical-psychoanalytic dialogue

Within Marx's framework, the capitalist and the proletariat are seen as political agents that embody the idea of enjoyment as a political factor. This idea, first introduced by Žižek in *For They Know Not What They Do* (1991), suggests that enjoyment as a political factor is not merely linked to ideological structures that rely on fantasy to obscure the disturbing realities facing the masses (Žižek, 2002b, p. 101). In a classic Lacanian sense, fantasy arises from the symbolic order, aiming to conceal the traumatic Real so that the masses can fetish and engage with the symbolic order with high satisfaction, without being disillusioned. It is widely accepted that the true role of ideology is to construct fantasies that enable people to indulge in the pleasure principle, thereby masking the obscene truths that disturb public consciousness (Jayanama, 2023, p. 56). In addition, Žižek's critical examination of enjoyment still raises a philosophical question about the ambiguity and mystical characteristics of human subjectivity: is humanity inherently rational and truly moral? (Žižek, 2002a, p. 220). Enjoyment can manifest as an individual's pursuit of actions that are disturbing and violate social and moral principles. Enjoyment is obtained by means of the subject's praxis in sacrificing the *telos* of the Good. This is why "we would sacrifice the good for the sake of enjoyment" (McGowan, 2013, p. 286). This pursuit of enjoyment, when embraced by the subject, can evolve into a political factor, its excessive behavior challenging the notions of rationality, calculation, mediocrity, morality, and virtue that are often collectively assumed by modern society.

The idea that enjoyment acts as a political factor permits a Lacanian-Marxist perspective on the politics of enjoyment, revealing a binary opposite forming a clear contrast within capitalism: the capitalist experiences and embraces enjoyment, while the proletariat is deprived of it. This approach seeks to seamlessly integrate Lacanian psychoanalysis with traditional Marxism, eliminating any potential for constructive disagreement between the two. This approach is ideological; psychoanalysis can empower traditional Marxism through three possible scenarios. First, capitalists experience enjoyment because they control and utilize the means of production – including land, resources, technologies, and capital. This enjoyment is tied to their ability to transform everything into a community oriented toward profit accumulation, consolidating their power both domestically as an oligarchy and internationally as imperialists: this troubling form of enjoyment undermines the rational and moral principles presupposed by modernity. Rather, it is the logic of capital that appears as the mystical image of the desire of the Other (Pavón-Cuéllar, 2024, p. 164). Second, the proletariat, regardless of racial, gender, or ethnic differences, is deprived of enjoyment because they do not possess the means of production. In this context, it can be asserted that capitalists have deprived the proletariat of enjoyment. Finally, the act of political emancipation or an epochal transition from capitalism to communism, led by a united global proletariat, symbolizes the proletariat's pursuit of reclaiming enjoyment from capitalists. In this communist vision, they can recuperate and retain a new mode of classless enjoyment: enjoyment based on the principle of egalitarianism. From these three scenarios, it is possible to conclude that the proletariat's reclamation of enjoyment forms harmony with Marx's notions of class struggle and class consciousness, which ultimately leads to the abolition of capitalism. This represents a classic teleological approach of Lacanian-Marxism. These scenarios illustrate the application of Lacanian enjoyment to support an old Left political framework – distinct from the Left-Laclauian populist paradigm – that is committed to opposing and abolishing capitalism.

In some respects, this idea of enjoyment as a political factor connects with Todd McGowan's conceptualization of two types of enjoyment within the politics of enjoyment. The first type is enjoyment associated with right-wing ideology, which McGowan refers to as "right-wing enjoyment". The right-wing enjoyment is characterized by an endless drive that supports the status quo, attacking perceived enemies to reinforce the existing phallic-power structures such as authoritarian regimes, oligarchies, imperialism, and populism to maintain a cohesiveness and totality of desire (McGowan, 2022, p. 42). Aligned with Marxist thought, this may refer to the enjoyment of the capitalist who acts as the oligarch at home (in Global North countries) and as the imperialist abroad (in Global South countries). The capitalist, believing that the world belongs to them, embodies and perpetuates right-wing enjoyment. In contrast, "left-wing enjoyment" represents enjoyment as a political factor within left-wing ideology. This type of enjoyment reflects a non-phallic enjoyment. It is experienced by those who feel excluded or alienated from the socio-economic systems created by capitalism. Soravis Jayanama entails McGowan's idea that the ontology of capitalism does not represent a phantasmatic wholeness; rather, it reveals an entanglement with lack, pain, and misery (Jayanama, 2022, p. 43). Ultimately, due to a shared sense of collective misery in the ontology of capitalism, these marginalized individuals seek to establish a space where people can gather, share, support one another, and engage in egalitarian principle.

In this space, although people are outsiders to one another and have different histories, stories, and narratives, they still manage to form intimate connections. Despite their differences, they no longer feel alienated; instead, they discover that they can create an external intimacy with each other (McGowan, 2022, pp. 7–9). This McGowanian space imaginary reflects what Lacan highlights as "extimacy", referring to something that the subject experienced as "the excluded in the interior" (Lacan as cited in Nadia Bou Ali and Surti Singh, 2025, p. 3). It is something external, strange, and bizarre that the subject intends to deny; however, it has always been an essential part of subjectivity from the beginning. McGowan's concept of extraordinarily particular space challenges capitalism and fosters constructive dissent among marginalized subjects, linked by the Lacanian notion of extimacy, contrasting sharply with Habermas's notion of a universal public sphere that seeks consensus among the social belonging and non-belonging members: in public sphere, "access is guaranteed to all citizens" (Habermas, 1974, p. 49). This McGowanian perspective implies universal Marxist anti-capitalism and critiques Laclauian radical democracy, which reduces anti-capitalism to a secondary political objective among the multiplication of antagonisms (Laclau and Mouffe, 2001, p. 192). Ultimately, Marxist politics highlight the solidarity of the proletariat across racial, gender, and national lines, emphasizing the need to recognize and resist various forms of capitalist exploitation. Nonetheless, a new society that aims to forge solidarity is at risk of giving rise to another form of false enjoyment in the dream of false egalitarianism (Žižek, 2022, p. 218).

Nonetheless, Lacan's exploration of enjoyment, as presented in his various seminars, reveals that enjoyment is also connected to other important psychoanalytic concepts such as masochism, sadism, narcissism, and, crucially, divine enjoyment. This connection is particularly evident in Lacan's critical discussions of women's desire, God's mystified enjoyment, and Antigone in Seminar VIII. In addition, Lacan's perspective on enjoyment creates both alignments and tensions with Marxism. This ambivalence in Lacanian psychoanalysis toward Marxism, especially the traditional Marxist, old Left paradigm, illustrates a divergence between Lacan's ideas and those of Marx. This ambivalence allows for a nuanced understanding that avoids oversimplifying Lacanian psychoanalysis as compatible with traditional Marxism.

Lacan's elaboration of enjoyment opens new avenues for understanding the proletariat in relation to various forms of enjoyment – such as masochism, sadism, narcissism, femininity, and divinity – coexisting within a single proletariat. This highlights how capitalism is maintained not solely through the capitalist's enjoyment but also through the proletariat's embodied experience of Lacanian enjoyment, which both supports capitalism and fuels resistance against it. Importantly, this indicates that each individual proletariat experiences a complex dialectic of enjoyment. A single proletariat may embody enjoyment that perpetuates capitalism – a pathological existence – while simultaneously experiencing enjoyment that aims to resist capitalism, akin to a woman's divine enjoyment rooted in the proletariat's subjectivity. This results in an internal contradiction of enjoyment, manifesting as an ontological tension for the proletariat. In essence, enjoyment does not operate within strict boundaries; its ontology resembles a Mobius strip. This complexity is often overlooked by Marx and traditional Marxism. This illustrates the utility of psychoanalysis in recognizing the limitations of Marxism, rather than uncritically applying it to support the politics of old Left Marxism.

Ultimately, this leads to a dialectic of proletariat self-enjoyment, making it increasingly difficult for the proletariat to distinguish between the types of enjoyment that sustain capitalism and those that seek to abolish it. The contradictory nature of enjoyment is inherent to the proletariat as a subject. At times, it reveals its unconscious desires through various paradoxical perspectives. In addition, it remains unclear about what it truly wants because it lacks a clear vision of historical change and is deprived of a convincing alternative future to the current status quo of capitalism. While there are some alternative futures or the possible tangible objectivities that focus on prospects like abundance and full automation, enjoyment itself does not necessitate a tangible object. The subject seeks enjoyment for its own sake. A notion reflects being-there rather than being as an end in itself: a dangerous political factor compared with a teleological notion like eudaimonia. It is important to recall Lacan's original definition of enjoyment: "when it speaks, it enjoys, and it knows nothing" (Lacan, 1999d, p. 104). This principle applies broadly to every subject that has embraced different political ideologies – whether right, left, centrist, or apathetic – until their circumstances are at risk of stagnation.

In conclusion, Marx's discussion of enjoyment within the capitalist mode of production reveals how capitalists develop excessive and addictive behaviors in their pursuit of enjoyment, while the proletariat is largely deprived of it. For the proletariat to reclaim enjoyment, a radical act of social transformation is necessary to achieve a new ideal of enjoyment known as classless enjoyment. This line of thought is somewhat linked to the idea of "enjoyment as a political factor", which suggests the division of enjoyment into "left" and "right" forms – manifested by the disenfranchised proletariat on one side and the capitalists, who feel a sense of ownership over the world, on the other. This chapter proposes an alternative perspective, suggesting that the proletariat experiences dialectical self-enjoyment, characterized by various forms of masochism, sadism, and narcissism. These elements inadvertently support the continuity of capitalism, resulting in a pathological condition of existence. However, there exists a form of divine enjoyment associated with the logic of the Lacanian Woman, representing feminine desire and the figure of Antigone. This divine enjoyment enables proletariat self-enjoyment to resist capitalism through acts of divine violence. This hybridization of God and Man is crucial for understanding proletariat subjectivity and revolutionary politics. Yet, enjoyment functions like a Mobius strip, creating an ontological rift in the proletariat's self-enjoyment. The enjoyment derived from revolutionary actions can be undermined by the enjoyment that perpetuates capitalism. This psychoanalytic dimension remains an overlooked aspect of Marx's thought and traditional Marxism.

Reference list

Ali, N. B., and Surti Singh. (2025). 'Introduction: The Concept of Extimacy', in *Extimacy*. Evanston: Northwestern University Press.

Castilla, E. (2025). 'The Meritocratic Ideal', in *The Meritocracy Paradox: Where Talent Management Strategies Go Wrong and How to Fix Them*. New York and West Sussex: Columbia University Press.

Freud, S. (2003). 'On the Introduction of Narcissism', in *Beyond the Pleasure Principle and Other Writings*. Translated by John Reddick. London: Penguin Books.

Habermas, J., Sara Lennox, and Frank Lennox. (1974). 'The Public Sphere: An Encyclopedia Article (1964)', *New German Critique* (Autumn), 49–55.

Holmstrom, N. (1981). 'Women's Work and Capitalism', *Science and Society*, 45(Summer).

Jayanama, S. (2023). 'Psychoanalysis, Politics, and Emancipation', in *Coz We are Lacking: The Politics of Enjoyment* [in Thai]. B&B Press: Bangkok.

Klein, M. (1975). 'On Observing the Behaviour of Young Infants (1952), in *Envy and Gratitude and Other Works 1946–1963*. New York: The Free Press.

Lacan, J. (1986). 'Translator's Note', in *The Seminar of Jacques Lacan Book XI: The Four Fundamental Concepts of Psychoanalysis*. Edited by Jacques-Alain Miller. Translated by Alan Sheridan. London: Penguin Books.

Lacan, J. (1999a) 'A Love Letter (*une lettre d'amour*)', in *The Seminar of Jacques Lacan Book XX: On Feminine Sexuality, The Limits of Love and Knowledge*. Edited by Jacques-Alain Miller. Translated by Bruce Fink. London and New York: W.W. Norton & Company.

Lacan, J. (1999b) 'God and Woman's Jouissance', in *The Seminar of Jacques Lacan Book XX: On Feminine Sexuality, The Limits of Love and Knowledge*. Edited by Jacques-Alain Miller. Translated by Bruce Fink. London and New York: W.W. Norton & Company.

Lacan, J. (1999c) 'On Jouissance', in *The Seminar of Jacques Lacan Book XX: On Feminine Sexuality, The Limits of Love and Knowledge*. Edited by Jacques-Alain Miller. Translated by Bruce Fink. London and New York: W.W. Norton & Company.

Lacan, J. (1999d) 'On the Baroque', in *The Seminar of Jacques Lacan Book XX: On Feminine Sexuality, The Limits of Love and Knowledge*. Edited by Jacques-Alain Miller. Translated by Bruce Fink. London and New York: W.W. Norton & Company.

Lacan, J. (2006a) 'A Theoretical Introduction to the Functions of Psychoanalysis in Criminology', in *Écrits: The First Complete Edition in English*. Translated by Bruce Fink. London and New York: W.W. Norton & Company.

Lacan, J. (2006b) 'Kant with Sade', in *Écrits: The First Complete Edition in English*. Translated by Bruce Fink. London and New York: W.W. Norton & Company.

Lacan, J. (2006c) 'Seminar on "The Purloined Letter"', in *Écrits: The First Complete Edition in English*. Translated by Bruce Fink. London and New York: W.W. Norton & Company.

Lacan, J. (2006d) 'The Freudian Thing or the Meaning of the Return to Freud in Psychoanalysis', in *Écrits: The First Complete Edition in English*. Translated by Bruce Fink. London and New York: W.W. Norton & Company.

Lacan, J. (2008a) 'Antigone Between Two Deaths', in *The Seminar of Jacques Lacan Book VII: The Ethics of Psychoanalysis*. Translated by Dennis Porter. New York and Oxon: Routledge.

Lacan, J. (2008b) 'The Articulations of the Play', in *The Seminar of Jacques Lacan Book VII: The Ethics of Psychoanalysis*. Translated by Dennis Porter. New York and Oxon: Routledge.

Lacan, J. (2008c) 'The Demand for Happiness and the Promise of Analysis', in *The Seminar of Jacques Lacan Book VII: The Ethics of Psychoanalysis*. Translated by Dennis Porter. New York and Oxon: Routledge.

Lacan, J. (2008d) 'The Function of the Good', in *The Seminar of Jacques Lacan Book VII: The Ethics of Psychoanalysis*. Translated by Dennis Porter. New York and Oxon: Routledge.

Lacan, J. (2008e) 'The *Jouissance* of Transgression', in *The Seminar of Jacques Lacan Book VII: The Ethics of Psychoanalysis*. Translated by Dennis Porter. New York and Oxon: Routledge.

Lacan, J. (2008f) 'The Paradoxes of Ethics or Have You Acted in Conformity with Your Desire', in *The Seminar of Jacques Lacan Book VII: The Ethics of Psychoanalysis*. Translated by Dennis Porter. New York and Oxon: Routledge.

Lacan, J. (2013). 'Can Psychoanalysis Constitute the Kind of Ethics Necessitated by our Times?', in *The Triumph of Religion*. Translated by Bruce Fink. Cambridge and Malden: Polity Press.

Lacan, J. (2021). 'Introduction', in *The Seminar of Jacques Lacan Book IV: The Object Relation*. Edited by Jacques Alain-Miller. Translated by A.R. Price. Cambridge and Medford: Polity Press.

Lacan, J. (2024a) 'From Surplus Value to Surplus *Jouissance*', in *The Seminar of Jacques Lacan Book XVI: From an Other to the Other*. Edited by Jacques Alain-Miller. Translated by Bruce Fink. Cambridge and Malford: Polity Press.

Lacan, J. (2024b) 'The One and Little a', in *The Seminar of Jacques Lacan Book XVI: From an Other to the Other*. Edited by Jacques Alain-Miller. Translated by Bruce Fink. Cambridge and Malford: Polity Press.

Laclau, E., and Chantal Mouffe. (2001). 'Hegemony and Radical Democracy', in *Hegemony and Socialist Strategy: Towards a Radical Democratic Politics*. 2nd Edition. London and New York: Verso.

Marx, K. (2004) 'Capital', in *Essential Thinkers: Karl Marx*. London: CRW Publishing Limited.

Marx, K. (2007). 'On the Jewish Question', in *Marx Early Political Writings*. Edited by Joseph O'Malley, and Richard Davis. Cambridge and New York: Cambridge University Press.

Marx, K. (2013). 'Machinery and Modern Industry', in *Karl Marx: Capital*. Edited by Tom Griffith. Hertfordshire: Wordsworth Editions Limited.

Marx, K. (2021). 'The Eighteenth Brumaire of Louis Bonaparte', in *Marx Later Political Writings*. Edited and Translated by Terrell Carver. Cambridge and New York: Cambridge University Press.

Marx, K. (2024). 'Wage, Labor, and Capital', in *The Communist Manifesto & Other Selected Writings*. London: William Collins Books.

Marx, K., and Friedrich Engels. (2004) 'Manifesto of the Communist Party', in *Essential Thinkers: Karl Marx*. London: CRW Publishing Limited.

McCarthy, P., and Marc Jones. (2005). 'Enjoyment in Youth Sport: Creating a Feel Good Factor', in *Psychology of Moods*. Edited by Anita Clark. New York: Nova Science Publishers.

McGowan, T. (2013). *Enjoying What We Don't Have: The Political Project of Psychoanalysis*. Lincoln and London: University of Nebraska Press.

McGowan, T. (2022). *Enjoyment Right & Left*. USA: Sublation Media.

Mitchell, S., and Margaret Black. (2016). 'Melanie Klein and Contemporary Kleinian Theory', in *Freud and Beyond*. New York: Basic Books.

Neuman, J., and Robert Baron. (2011). 'Social Antecedents of Bullying: A Social Interactionist Perspective', in *Bullying and Harassment in the Workplace: Developments in Theory, Research, and Practice*. 2nd Edition. Edited by Ståle Einarsen, Helge Hoel, Dieter Zapf, and Cary L. Cooper. London and New York: CRC Press.

Novara Media. (2025). 'The REAL Point of Trump's Tariffs | Aaron Bastani Meets Slavoj Žižek', April 13, 2025. https://www.youtube.com/watch?v=mw5zZw4yUIc. Accessed: December 30, 2025.

Pavón-Cuéllar, D. (2024). 'The Jouissance of Capital: Noted for a Lacanian Critique of Political Economy', in *Political Jouissance*. Edited by Nicol A. Barria-Asenjo, and Slavoj Žižek. London and New York: Bloomsbury Academic.

Sontag, S. (2003). *Regarding the Pain of Others*. New York: Picador.

The Institute of Art and Ideas (2025). 'What is the true nature of the Self? | Slavoj Žižek, Carlo Rovelli, Alenka Zupančič'. December 20, 2025. 15:52 min. https://www.youtube.com/watch?v=DbUatLXVq4c. Accessed: December 29, 2025.

Weber, M. (2001). 'Asceticism and the Spirit of Capitalism', in *The Protestant Ethic and the Spirit of Capitalism*. Translated by Talcott Parsons. London and New York: Routledge

Weinbaum, B. (1978). *The Curious Courtship of Women's Liberation and Socialism*. South End Press.

Young, M. (2008). *The Rise of the Meritocracy*. London and New Brunswick: Transaction Publishers.

Žižek, S. (2000). 'The Hegelian Ticklish Subject', in *The Ticklish Subject: The Absent Centre of Political Ontology*. London and New York: Verso.

Žižek, S. (2002a). 'All's Well that Ends Well?', in *For they know not what they do: Enjoyment as a Political Factor*. 2nd Edition. London and New York: Verso.

Žižek, S. (2002b). 'Hegelian Llangue', in *For they know not what they do: Enjoyment as a Political Factor*. 2nd Edition. London and New York: Verso.

Žižek, S. (2008). 'Divine Violence", in *Violence: Six Sideways Reflections*. New York: Picador.

Žižek, S. (2022). 'Surplus-Enjoyment, Or, Why Do We Enjoy Our Oppression', in *Surplus-Enjoyment*. London and New York: Bloomsbury.

Žižek, S. (2024). '"If there is a god, then anything is permitted": On Dostoevsky, freedom, and religious violence', *ABC*, January 22, 2024. https://www.abc.net.au/religion/slavoj-zizek-if-there-is-a-god-then-anything-is-permitted/10100616. Accessed: December 30, 2025.

Žižek, S. (2025). 'Worlds Blown into Space', in *Zero Point*. London and New York: Bloomsbury.

6 Reassessing surplus-value

Proletariat in the two dimensions of anxiety and a psychoanalytic act

This chapter aims to reassess Karl Marx's concept of surplus-value – the relationship between the proletariat as a human asset in the mode of production governed by capitalism, resulting in the existential surplus of the commodity at the expense of the unfair rate of wage and payment to the proletariat. Surplus-value is defined as the proletariat's relationship to capitalism. In a Lacanian perspective, surplus-value is a signifier not only of the proletariat experiencing exploitation but also of the capitalist's surplus-enjoyment. It is the underpinning capitalist subjective surplus-enjoyment that is capable of letting capitalism as an objective surplus-enjoyment, pertaining to a dominant framework where social relationship between man, capital, exploitation, commodity, and profit is mutually engaged in a transcendental reproduction of this reality, where an attempt to forever fulfill a lack of desire is at stake. For an amalgamation between Marx and Jacques Lacan, discussing surplus-value with surplus-enjoyment – how the two terms form conceptual linkages and deviations – seems to be an absolute closure, in other words, it is apparently a confinement. Against this absolute closure, it remains possible for another Lacanian significant notion, such as anxiety, to create an ontological gap, an epistemic rethinking, and offer an alternative perspective regarding Marx's surplus-value. Significantly, departing from connecting surplus-value with surplus-enjoyment, this chapter highlights that surplus-value is linked to Lacan's conception of anxiety.

Based on the four fundamental dimensions of the proposed proletariat discourse – psyche, existence, subject, and politics – this chapter proceeds in four sections. Resorting to Lacan's original source, Seminar X entitled "Anxiety", the first section contradicts a Gestalt of anxiety, believing that anxiety occurs in the absence of the object. Lacan rather highlights the emergence of anxiety in relation to the presence of the object. Following Hegelian dialectic, Lacan suggests anxiety is twofold. First, anxiety is related to the desire of the Other; the subject complies with the desire of the Other – the Other's *jouissance* – in order to manage the anxiety of alienation and the feeling of non-belonging. Second, anxiety is linked to the subject's refusal to compromise with the desire of the Other, particularly in relation to how the Other expects the subject to align with its desires.

DOI: 10.4324/9781003657781-6

Paradoxically, when the subject seeks something beyond the desires that the Other assumes, this object cause of desire – often referred to as *objet a* – tends to betray the subject, like the precious thing that the subject yearning for turns out to be the object of death and annihilation: a dimensionality that is addressed by Lacan in 1962–1963 in his departure from his articulation of *objet a* in his earlier works. This circumstance requires attention to Lacan's notions of stupidity, in which the subject is let down and does not get up, and certainty, in which the subject is let down and gets up in the midst of pain, agony, and disappointment. These two aspects of anxiety are vital for unravelling traditional Marxism's limitations on the proletariat's relationship to capitalism and communism.

In the second section, it argues that surplus-value is the proletariat's means of existence and to ward off the cloud of anxiety disturbing their mind. Paradoxically, this proletariat's consent to exist as a surplus-value may dismantle the necessity to separate from the existing situation and a defiance of capitalism. The third section introduces Lacan's elaboration of psychoanalytic Act, comprised of *passage à l'acte* and acting-out, embodied by the subject, including the proletariat subject, the subject that opposes and liberates themselves from being reduced as the surplus-value in relation to existence and anxiety. The proletariat subject may develop a phantasmatic thinking that the world after capitalism is better than the current being, but the law of *objet a* suggests on the contrary that it is probably not. It becomes a huge question for the proletariat subject and how they form a subjective relationship to the objective existence that fails them. If they continue a psychoanalytic Act as acting-out, then this proletariat subject can be understood as a subject of certainty. But if they continue a psychoanalytic Act as *passage à l'acte*, then this proletariat subject is inclined toward a subject of stupidity, unless they sublimate from stupidity to certainty, in the midst of pain that the *objet a* is the object cause of doubt for the subject, whether this object is really a cause of desire or not. The fourth section brings Lacan's articulation on the two aspects of anxiety in relation to psychoanalytic Act to engage with the contemporary Marxist notion entitled degrowth communism, in order to portray its limitation, arguing that degrowth communism is probably the *objet a* – a cause of desire, betrayal, and doubt – and the Marxist subject who wishes to maintain it is encouraged to be the subject of certainty, negating themselves as the signifier of stupidity.

The two dimensions of Lacanian anxiety: anxiety, dialectic, and the psyche

In general psychology, anxiety is often described as the tension experienced by an individual in relation to their unacknowledged fears, without the presence of specific objects or triggers. In simpler terms, the Gestalt of anxiety is understood as an imperative part of the subject's experience that occurs independently of any external object. However, Lacan's psychoanalytic perspective challenges this notion. Lacan asserts that "it is wrong to say that anxiety is without object" (Lacan, 2014k, p. 76). According to Lacan, the essence of anxiety is indeed "not without object" (Lacan, 2014m, p. 100).

The term "object" is inherently dialectical, encompassing two levels of meaning. The first level pertains to the Other – specifically, the big Other or *i* (a) – which is linked to the symbolic order and plays a role in forming the barred subject ($), resulting in a false ego-consciousness. The second level refers to the *objet a*, or the small object a or *i'* (a), where the subject begins to question the integrity of their ego-consciousness, driven by the Other, while seeking a lost object beyond the confines of the symbolic order. This distinction between the Other and the certain type of object, the *objet a*, highlights the otherness of something that does not prevail in the signifying field of the Other. Understanding the object at these two levels prompts Lacan's methodological approach to anxiety, utilizing Hegelian dialectical methods. He asserts, "We are going to see the function of anxiety being introduced into the play of dialectic that knots these two levels so tightly together" (Lacan, 2014a, p. 6).

Therefore, regarding the principle of Hegelian dialectic as it applies to the object as the Other and as *objet a*, Lacan's understanding of anxiety encompasses two dimensions as follows.

The first dimension of anxiety: the other, desire, jouissance, and fantasy

In the first dimension, the concept of anxiety as described by Lacan explores the relationship between the formation of a subject's question of desire and the response from the desire of the Other. Lacan states that "before knowing what my relation to its desire means when I am in a state of anxiety, I put this Other here, capital A" (Lacan, 2014b, p. 22). He further emphasizes, "As I told you, man's desire is the desire of the Other" (Lacan, 2014b, p. 22). Based on this relationship with the Other, the subject lacks enjoyment but can feel either safe or insulated from experiencing anxiety, particularly when there is a consistent relationship of homogeneity among the subject, desire, and the Other.

Anxiety arises in the psyche of the subject when a previously smooth relationship becomes disrupted. This anxiety can occur when the subject seeks recognition or acknowledgment from the Other, but the Other refuses to acknowledge the subject's existence. When the Other deprives the subject of their desires, it can lead to a form of self-fragmentation experienced by the subject. When the subject is dependent on the Other, anxiety occurs as a result of the subject neglected by the Other, which means that feelings of neglect can make the subject feel as though their entire world is collapsing. This neglect triggers unconscious mechanisms that ultimately lead to the experience of anxiety.

This dynamic occurs because various subjects, such as the proletariat, grapple with a profound question regarding their lack of desire and the loss of a unified self. To fill this void, which contributes to their anxiety, they agree to be used as human labor force as surplus-value by their employers and capitalist leaders. This reliance on the desires of the Other helps the proletariat alleviate some of their anxiety. In Lacan's thesis, the following logic will serve as a subject's scenario of anxiety-experience. Since the subject's desire depends on the Other, this gives rise to dual postulation. For the first postulation, the Other is a locus of ego-consciousness formulation of the subject. For the second, the Other is always gazing upon and monitoring the subject. Lacan explains,

> I will say right off, to make you feel what is at issue, that in Hegel, concerning the dependence of my desire with respect to the desirer who is the Other, I am dealing in the most certain and articulated way with the Other as consciousness. The Other is the one who sees me.
>
> (Lacan, 2014b, p. 23)

This means that a subject experiencing anxiety attacks may choose to cooperate with the Other, which aids in developing their ego-consciousness, understanding their lack of desire, and providing necessary support: the Other becomes the answer to the subject's lack of desire. While seeking relief from anxiety through the symbolic field of desire called the Other, the subject represents a "barred subject" ($), losing aspects of their true self.

Discussing anxiety in the first dimension requires a comparison between anxiety and fantasy. Lacan notes that the structure of anxiety is not far from fantasy (Lacan, 2014a, p. 3). He aims to clarify the meaning of anxiety by highlighting that the subject exists in the space between their own desires and the desire of the Other. The desire of the Other shows a signifier of *jouissance* that belongs to the Other: it is not the subject's *jouissance*. As Lacan states, "this is where anxiety is situated" – in the gap between desire and *jouissance* (Lacan, 2014d, p. 175). The subject's desire pertains to an individual's personal longing, particularly their will for *jouissance*. While the English translation of *jouissance* is "enjoyment", Lacan's instruction in Seminar X suggests that the term "encompasses" a range of meanings. Beyond simply enjoyment, *jouissance* relates to the subject's sublimation that emerged from the rim-structure of the circle of reality. It refers to the subject in search of the cause of desire, excess, and can also imply an active pursuit of a lost object, often leading to pain, tragedy, agony, and self-destruction experienced by the subject. Understanding the term *jouissance* properly requires examining from the perspective of the subject, as well as from the perspective of the Other.

From the perspective of the subject, *jouissance* involves the subject's quest for something beyond the limitations of the symbolic order, driven by a desire for what is missing – like the revolutionary proletariat seeking a communist world unattainable in a capitalist context. For such subjects, the symbolic order becomes a representation of lack and incompleteness regarding their desires. Here, *jouissance* is thus linked to a desire that exceeds the desire of the Other, as the revolutionary subject seeks the elusive *objet a* – in this case, a communist world – an excessive object that eludes an existing symbolic signification. According to Lacan, the *objet a* is seen to resist a universal signifier of desire. He states that "any assimilation to the function of a signifier and this indeed is why it symbolizes that which, in the sphere of the signifier, always presents itself as lost, as what gets lost in signifierization" (Lacan, 2014d, p. 174). Lacan continues *objet a* as the object forming a cause of desire on a condition that it is "an object that is external to any possible definition of objectivity" (Lacan, 2014h, p. 86). But whether the subject's search for this lost object will be successful is a different question altogether.

From the perspective of the Other, *jouissance* is tied to the desire of the Other. The subject often compromises to fulfill the Other's demand, which means that the subject is seeking recognition from the Other to alleviate anxiety. By aligning their own desires with the Other, they risk becoming a perverse figure or extreme masochist, binding themselves to the Other's transcendentalism of desire. This compliance aims to gain recognition within the symbolic order, which helps prevent anxiety. This willingness to conform to the desire of the Other leads the subject's choice of freewill to instrumentalize their own life for the *jouissance* of the Other, often as a way to compensate for something lacking. In other words, by complying with the desire of the Other, the subject seeks full acknowledgment in the symbolic order, which acts as the most effective means of preventing anxiety attacks. As a result, the subject often forgets and dismisses the critical reflection that the *jouissance* of the Other, which they embrace, is actually a fantasy.

Lacan critiques this fantasy of anxiety-erasure developed by the subject, believing that it is difficult for the subject to withdraw from this fetishism, asserting that "this is why I am saying that targeting the Other's *jouissance* is a fantasmatic target" (Lacan, 2014c, p. 163). Lacan's criticism points out the problematic nature of the subject's reliance on the desire of the Other to manage anxiety. He warns that there is something "more" involved; this something "more" emphasizes the aspect of the subject that is fallen away, far away from the subject's relation to the Other's *jouissance*, this non-relationship in the subject is typical when confronting an aspect of the subject that is more essential than any other part of themselves (Lacan, 2014c, p. 167).

The barred subject begins searching for something more – something irreducible that lies outside the desire of the Other. This implies that there is a remainder (Lacan, 2014d, p. 174) that exists independently of the structure of fantasy related to the Other. In Lacan's own terms, this "$ desire of *a*" (Lacan, 2014m, p. 100) represents the subject's quest for a lost object. This subject is separate from the realm of the Other; it represents another dimension of the object of desire, which involves a disconnection from the subject that feels lost and alienated within the fantasy.

Nonetheless, a key aspect to consider is that the subject's desire to connect with the *objet a* may not lead to personal fulfillment, happiness, or overwhelming joy. Instead, this pursuit often brings about a different kind of anxiety. According to Lacan, anxiety is linked to the *objet a*, as he explains that "it is also, paradoxically, the level at which the object *a* is most fully masked and at which, by virtue of this fact, the subject is most assured in relation to anxiety" (Lacan, 2014f, p. 325).

The second dimension of anxiety: **objet a**, *stupidity, and certainty*

In contrast to the first dimension, anxiety in the second dimension begins with Lacan's emphasis on *objet a* – the object as forming a non-relationship and a fallen away from the desire of the Other – which is a reminiscence of *niederfallen* (fallen away) according to Freud's neologism. Lacan states, "This object a whose constituent characteristics we have merely touched on and which today we are putting on the agenda, is what is in question whenever Freud speaks about the object in connection with anxiety" (Lacan, 2014g, p. 40). To understand the radical aspect of the subject's anxiety, it is essential to consider both a Freudian perspective and a point of Hegelian dialectic as adopted by Lacan. The presence of the Other allows the subject to alleviate anxiety. However, concerning the concept of the *objet a*, anxiety arises not just as the source of desire and the irreducible remainder but also because, as the subject strives to approach and even possess the *objet a*, nothing ultimately manifests. A Hegelian dialectic adopted by Lacan allows him to say that the object of desire is possible, meaning that the subject can reach, possess, touch, and grab it firmly, only insofar as such object of desire becomes none. Lacan clarifies this by stating, "I shall simply tell you that, at the level of *i' (a)*, which is the *virtual image* of a *real image*, nothing appears" (Lacan, 2014g, p. 40; italics in the original). When the subject finally realizes that at the apex of their relationship with the phantasmatic object that they are yearning for, their object of desire is empty or lacking substance, anxiety emerges due to the fear of losing their enjoyment. This fear drives them to continually repeat the same mistaken act, hoping to discover a different object that will bring them enjoyment; however, this quest for enjoyment may ultimately be unachievable.

The concept of the object of desire is shaped by a reality principle that distinguishes between permissible and prohibited objects. However, the lost object, which represents the object of desire as defined by the subject, challenges this principle because it is neither entirely acceptable nor entirely forbidden; it is the excess or something that is beyond the reality principle. The lost object refers to something that the subject once possessed but has since been separated from due to the constraints of reality, leading to a subject searching and re-searching for it. When this object is encountered again, it is essential to understand that it is not the same as what was originally lost. This realization initiates a dialectical process. As Lacan observes, "the object of the first weaning found again . . . is not the same object and will never be", highlighting that "what is sought out is never sought out in the same way as what will be found" (Lacan, 2021, p. 7): threatening the subject to be deprived of enjoyment.

This image of *objet a* offers a different perspective from the traditional understanding based on Lacan's demonstration of the ontological tension between the subject, drive, and *objet a*. In the traditional view established in 1960, Lacan identifies the concept of *objet a* as the object that carries a "minus sign" or is referred to as "agalma" – the precious leftover in the subject (Lacan, 2006, p. 699). This object remains hidden from the desire of the Other, which plays a crucial role in shaping the subject's fantasy, informing what they should desire. However, when this fantasy is traversed, the responsibility of the *objet a* intensifies, leading to a deep and often violent division within the subject. This means that, initially, in the first step, the subject must keep this object of desire to themselves, as they cannot attain it in reality. Furthermore, in the second step, it is this sense of lack that drives the subject to sublimate their identities, transforming themselves into something else, to live on, and thereby becoming distanced from the object of desire that now becomes forever the object of lost or impossibility. For example, in Lacan's view, the penis serves as the object of desire for women (Lacan, 2006, p. 699). This situation leads to third significant consequences: first, women cannot possess this object in reality; second, they may sublimate themselves as if to embody the phallus – the leftover – seeking to dominate others such as their boyfriends as if they embody masculinity; third, penis as a representation of the object of woman's desire appears to be the impossible and lost forever. In other words, in this conventional view, a subject driven by a desire for an object causes frustration and irritation because this object is always dismissed and deferred from catching it. In this scenario, the *objet a* is the impossible object, and the subject's active drive is ultimately in vain and exhausting. The subject, circulating around the object of desire without being able to possess, master, or consume it, is reduced to being merely a naked drive. This leads to suffering and self-fragmentation for the subject in the end.

However, Lacan's evolution of the concept of *objet a* leads to another crucial question: what happens when a subject has an opportunity to connect directly with the *objet a*, even to catch it? Lacan's response in 1962–1963, especially in Seminar X is even more radical: "nothing appears" in the *objet a*, as mentioned earlier. This is because the object that causes desire will ultimately betray the subject, failing to align with their imagination and completely disappointing their expectations. Lacan emphasizes the role of the *objet a* as a transitional element in understanding desire. This concept illustrates the shift from the object that ignites the cause of desire to the object that ultimately disappoints the subject. Lacan (2014i) describes this as the object "that which deceives not" (p. 312), highlighting its intrinsic quality of void and nothingness within the object itself.

It is more critical and crucial to understand that *objet a* ultimately represents itself as a truth for the subject that its precedent ontology is marked by affection fueled with an obscenity, creating a distance between the subject and the object.

Anxiety manifests phenomenally because, after an extensive search, the subject comes to realize that the real image of the *objet a* is no longer an object of desire but rather a source of betrayal, affecting the subject: this is why Lacan emphasizes that "anxiety is an affect" (Lacan, 2014a, pp. 14–15). This realization leads to a relapse, leaving the subject in a state of lacking desire. Lacan articulates this point clearly: "At this level, you are *a*, the object, and everyone knows that this is what is intolerable – not only to discourse itself, which, after all, betrays this" (Lacan, 2014m, p. 103).

The presence of *objet a* indicates that this object ceases to be a straightforward cause of desire or enjoyment but which in turn generates a genuine cause of anxiety. This anxiety represents a fear of failure and collapse, replacing potential enjoyment derived from the object. In these structures, anxiety reveals its fundamental connection to the object as a failure. Its primary role is to serve as a leftover of the subject, the "subject as real" (Lacan, 2014c, p. 165). Specific to the context in Seminar X, the "subject as real" does not imply the subject's ideological resistance to the symbolic order. Instead, it suggests that trying to establish a connection with *objet a* is inherently a failure. Even when the subject finally grasps, catches, and touches the *objet a*, they are paradoxically left with a sense of lack, deprived of enjoyment, as if the object has slipped through their fingers. At the level of *objet a* as the real, "what is called upon there is unable to appear there" (Anxiety, 2014e, p. 45). The process in which desire seems to manifest as fulfillment ultimately exposes itself as an absence. This explains why anxiety is linked to *objet a* and affect; it is paradoxically an object that appears yet simultaneously disappears from the subject's grasp, and this largely affects the subject's entire realm of psyche.

To understand Lacan's conception of anxiety, one must recognize his dependence on Hegel's philosophy. Following Hegel, Lacan represents the metaphor of the *objet a* with "a glove turned inside out" (Lacan, 2014l, p. 66), highlighting how the subject's desire attempts to invert this glove. However, elements within the glove resist this inversion, suggesting that the subject is eager to turn it inside out. This signifies a connection between the subject and the *objet a*, yet in the real, the object resists the subject's efforts, the subject's enjoyment is taken away, causing significant anxiety to the subject. The transformation of the *objet a* from absent to present does not yield lasting fulfillment. Importantly, the *objet a* is not entirely unreachable; the subject's ability to connect with it at its real level implies that "its ultimate mainspring may elude him indefinitely" (Lacan, 2014l, p. 66). The object's resistance to being inverted or possessed causes anxiety in relation to the present object. The *objet a*, according to Lacan, represents "that which deceives not" at the level of the real (Lacan, 2014k, p. 76). It can be metaphorically described as a book that appears open but ultimately turns out to be "a closed book on the subject" (Lacan, 2014k, p. 76). Another metaphor likens the *objet a* to a letter that reaches its intended destination. Although the letter is opened, it reveals itself to be "the unopened letters sending him off again under closed seal to further traces" (Lacan, 2014k, p. 76), which forces the subject to question their own desire once more.

Anxiety is linked to a subject's sense of inadequacy. This connection arises because "anxiety is not without object" (Lacan, 2014k, p. 76). While anxiety can deceive the subject, it also compels the individual to revisit their own desires and, at times, to question those desires. Consequently, anxiety emerges when the *objet a* associated with the subject becomes a "cause of doubt" (Lacan, 2014k, p. 76), highlighting the subject's feeling of inadequacy and the desire as vacuity and emptiness even though at the stage where the subject is linked with the *objet a*, which ultimately thwarts and betrays their quest for fulfillment, leading the subject to re-experience a sense of lack. This gives rise to stupidity. Stupidity, in this context, is not merely the subject's inability to exert influence or assert a dominant voice within the symbolic order; it also encompasses the subject's relentless search for the new object cause of desire, after the feeling of betrayal, which can result again in self-destructive act and a profound sense of failure. In other words, stupidity results from a subject's disappointment with the *objet a* but remains an active drive that is constantly misled by another illusory object cause of desire without cutting this toxic loop. After encountering disappointment, the subject of stupidity will look for a new object of desire, anticipating that it will fulfill a totality of desire to the subject, and they will fail even more.

However, in Lacan, it is not enough to end all discussions at the level of subject and stupidity. This furthermore requires the subject to transform stupidity into certainty. For the idea of certainty, this does not refer to the subject's absolute domination in the symbolic order. Certainty does not mean the subject's completion of himself as a total signifier. Instead, certainty is related to the subject and the act, namely the act that is caught in the cycle of being dropped and then getting up. It is implicit in Lacan's teaching that a subject in transforming stupidity to certainty is a signifier of the subject, which is "*letting oneself drop and getting up on the stage*" (Lacan, 2014j, p. 114, italics in the original). The characteristic of the subject, in terms of certainty, refers to a person who seeks an object of desire, even though that object does not bring them complete satisfaction. They feel compelled to maintain their desire, which is fundamentally rooted in a sense and perception of lack, in order to prevent it from becoming a lost object. Essentially, they are compelled to find enjoyment in this desire, despite it being characterized as lack. Anxiety arises not because the object of desire fails to provide total fulfillment but because the object, defined by its lack, is at risk of being perceived as a complete loss. The presence of something that is ultimately unsatisfactory is preferable to having nothing at all. Paradoxically, the object of desire is tied to the subject through this sense and perception of lack, yet the subject needs to accept and embrace it as a source of enjoyment, all while guarding it from being lost. If the desire characterized as a lack is lost, anxiety will ensue.

To combat anxiety, the subject – viewed as a signifier of certainty – must engage in a repetitive cycle where the object of desire is constantly at risk of faltering. Although desire signifies lack and reflects deficiency, the subject as certainty must preserve it as a source of enjoyment, even embracing such dissatisfaction and displeasure emanated from the object. This situation is intrinsic to the subject's role as a signifier of certainty.

A dialogue with traditional Marxism: anxiety, stupidity, and certainty

The Lacanian discussion on stupidity and certainty is significant for both traditional Marxism and its revolutionary perspectives, as these perspectives are often constrained by class consciousness while neglecting critical issues raised by the psychoanalytic approach. Ultimately, what the proletariat needs most in this context is a Lacanian understanding of stupidity and certainty, rather than a fantasy of communist utopianism based on the concept of totality and a traditional Marxist interpretation of history through the lens of commodity fetishism, which is believed to give birth to universal class consciousness. From a Lacanian perspective, there are two main points to consider.

First, Lacan's concept of stupidity suggests that, rather than focusing solely on class consciousness, the proletariat and its vision for global revolution may become trapped in a repetitive cycle of rising and falling throughout history. Victories may be viewed as betrayals, leading the proletariat, after experiencing disappointments, to repeatedly engage in acts of revolution – often resulting in failure – until such failures reach a transcendental level. The Lacanian concept of stupidity raised awareness against traditional Marxism, which can be understood as fail again, fail even more. This idea contrasts with the phrase "fail again, fail better", which may be perceived as a Marxist fantasy, illustrating that the proletariat, as a revolutionary force, will ultimately save everyone – despite their failures today, they will succeed tomorrow.

Second, Lacan's concept of certainty aligns with Hegel's well-known assertion that "history repeats itself, first as tragedy, then as farce". This Lacanian interpretation of certainty offers an alternative view to the traditional Marxist understanding of the proletariat. It warns against the complacency that can arise from solely achieving class consciousness, which can foster the belief that this Marxist metaphysical consciousness will magically lead to a proletariat revolution that abolishes capitalism and ushers in a communist society. Such a linear perspective on history is a fantasy of traditional Marxism regarding the proletariat and the communist world. While striving for class consciousness, the proletariat aims for revolution with its immense force and global solidarity, but this approach overlooks issues of racial discrimination, gender discrimination, and national prejudice that exist among them: global solidarity, as endorsed by traditional Marxism, signifies a lack of egalitarian enjoyment.

At this point, it is not necessary for anyone to shift from traditional Marxism – specifically Western Marxism – in order to engage with the challenges and historical contexts of non-Western countries and foster dialogue with non-Western and post-colonial Marxism. Proponents of Western Marxism may assume that studying non-Western Marxism provides an opportunity to confront its own limitations and improve its theoretical framework. However, this perspective overlooks the possibility and positionality that Lacanian psychoanalysis – a Western knowledge and theory – can help traditional Marxism recognize its limitations and enhance its theories from within, without having to rely on non-Western and post-colonial Marxism for such insight.

Everything hinges on how Marxism interacts with psychoanalysis. How does Marxism situate Lacanian psychoanalysis? It is suggested that psychoanalysis should avoid aligning itself with Marxism without acknowledging any inconsistencies or conflicts between the two. Instead of merely using psychoanalysis to bolster Marxism without engaging in constructive dialogue and argument, psychoanalysis should also be permitted as a critique of Marxism. This approach can ultimately contribute to the improvement of Marxism, and this informs why Marxism needs psychoanalysis. For instance, psychoanalysis argues that a traditional Marxist fantasy overlooks the psychoanalytic implications of Lacanian anxiety, suggesting that the communist world may represent another form of the castration of enjoyment, and, hence, the communist world becomes an object of betrayal for the proletariat. Furthermore, the idea of Lacanian certainty implies that a communist world would be one overwhelmed by the unresolved challenges known as the Real faced by the proletariat. The communist world would likely be a signifier that embodied a lack of desire. This highlights that the shift from tragedy to farce emphasizes not the idealistic elements of communist utopianism but the critical need for the proletariat to preserve their fragile communist world from destruction, preventing it from becoming a lost cause.

Existence: reassessing Marx's surplus-value as a Lacanian anxiety

Exploring Marx's surplus-value

Instead of defining philosophy as a separate endeavor from interpreting the world to support ideological movements aimed at changing it, it can be said that the task of philosophy for the proletariat is to interpret existence itself. This understanding of Being has to be prioritized to eventually separate from the world, a concept that resonates with Lacan's neologism "ex-sistence", a notion that is laced with a negation of the subject from the existing ground of being. Before attempting to change the world, it is essential to thoroughly understand it as it actually is. Changing the world without this critical interpretation can lead to painful and misguided transformations in society. Many theories and social movements fail because they attempt to alter the world without first comprehending it. Following their failures and the resulting suffering, they often need to return to the task of interpreting the world. Thus, philosophy is crucial for the proletariat as a means of interpreting the world independently before seeking to change it. In this light, it is realized that Marx's concept of surplus-value is not merely a question regarding a relation of production but a mode of self-inquiry, which Marx offers to the proletariat. Surplus-value is not the philosophy of changing the world, but it represents the movement of interpreting the world surrounding the proletariat prior to any attempts to transform it.

This section will reassess Marx's concept of surplus-value in relation to the proletariat, specifically through a Lacanian psychoanalytic perspective imposed on Marx's *Theories of Surplus-Value*. This analysis reveals that Marx's notion of surplus-value is connected to Lacan's discussions on anxiety. Surplus-value can be understood as a mechanism through which the proletariat attempts to alleviate anxiety and prevent anxiety attacks. Rather than simply comparing Marx's surplus-value with Lacan's idea of surplus-enjoyment, the argument in this section posits that the proletariat's voluntary engagement as a surplus-value serves as a coping strategy to manage anxiety and the feeling of alienation within a capitalist society. This perspective also sheds light on why the proletariat may abandon class consciousness and consent to capitalist realism, despite grappling with mental health issues, burnout, and unproductive work (Fisher, 2009, p. 73; Graber, 2018, p. 101). A significant yet often overlooked aspect of discussions on capitalist realism is the proletariat's active-masochistic choice to engage with a repressive regime mode of production called surplus-value, which they use as a means to combat feelings of alienation and ultimately reduce anxiety.

Based on Marx's original insights, he explains surplus-value in *Theories of Surplus-Value, Part I*. Surplus-value refers to the additional value generated from the proletariat's labor that exceeds the wages they receive. According to Marx, understanding surplus-value requires considering four key factors: (a) the proletariat as the labor force, (b) a commodity, (c) the labor time involved, and (d) wages. Surplus-value highlights the injustices inherent in the economic system. It arises when the proletariat invests labor time and effort to produce a commodity but receives compensation through wages that are unequal to the time and effort expended in the production process. A paradox is that any labor generating surplus-value is highly praised from a capitalist standpoint as productive labor, which can lead the proletariat to believe they are contributing meaningfully through their work, even though this type of work is often unproductive and can result in burnout. The proletariat participates in this regime because it provides them with a sense of belonging, functioning similarly to therapy by alleviating their anxiety. Marx defines surplus-value from the perspective of capitalist production as labor power that produces a value greater than its own cost (Marx, 1975a, p. 152). In this sense, equality can be defined as any proletariat whose investment of labor power equals the rate of wage return and the time spent working. However, the capitalist system disrupts this equality because, as Marx states, "in the capitalist sense it would not be productive because it produced no surplus value" (Marx, 1975a, p. 153).

In *Theories of Surplus-Value, Part II*, Marx describes surplus-value as "the excess of value of the product *over* the value of the wages" (Marx, 1975b, p. 406; original italics). For surplus-value to emerge, the proletariat must first be compelled to work beyond the necessary time, and this compulsion is exerted by capital (Marx, 1975b, p. 406). In Part III of *Theories of Surplus-Value*, Marx links the origin of surplus-value to the employment of an excessive quantity of labor within a capitalist framework. He defines the proletariat as unpaid laborers. Surplus-value represents capitalism's utilization of "the surplus quantity of living labor, for which it is exchanged as the source of profit" (Marx, 1975c, p. 15). It refers to the significant amount of living labor that goes into the production process. The proletariat works to sustain this process for the profit of the capitalist yet receives no equivalent payment in return. Thus, the proletariat becomes "the unpaid labor which capital appropriates in this pseudo-exchange" (Marx, 1975c, p. 15).

In his critique of David Ricardo's theory of profit, Marx argues that both Ricardo and John Stuart Mill, a supporter of Ricardo's ideas, fail to recognize that profit is not solely determined by the value of the commodity, a reduction in production costs due to machinery replacing human labor, or customer demand for specific products. For Marx, profit is fundamentally tied to the labor time that the proletariat invests in the commodity, which is owned by the capitalist. While this ownership is established through legal means, such as a work contract, it becomes questionable when considering that the labor time, like working days, is often inadequately compensated. According to Marx, surplus-value "depends not only on the rate at which the surplus labor of the individual worker is appropriated but likewise on the number of workers exploited at the same time" (Marx, 1975c, p. 191).

Reassessing Marx's surplus-value in the first dimension of anxiety

It is observed that referring closely to Marx's original sources – the *Theories of Surplus Value*, Parts 1, 2, and 3 – surplus-value represents a scenario of injustice rooted in the labor exploitation inherent in capitalism. Marx's concept of surplus-value is connected to the productive labor power utilized as part of the means of production. This results in structural class conflict within the workplace, arising from the time worked beyond what is necessary, as stipulated in the employment contract, which is exerted by the capitalist. From the capitalist's perspective, every unit of productive labor power has to generate surplus-value. Consequently, this situation perpetuates itself, as the surplus labor of the proletariat is appropriated and integrated into the production process without receiving a fair rate of compensation.

Rejecting the capitalist framework could lead to a loss of existence, prompting the proletariat to actively cooperate with their freewill as a surplus-value, not for the sake of surplus-enjoyment for themselves but for the proletariat's existential fulfillment. This viewpoint contradicts Marxist humanism's belief that capitalism dehumanizes the proletariat. Marx argues that while the proletariat's utility in production exists, it is not deemed productive in a capitalist sense because it does not generate surplus-value. He notes that capitalist productivity relies on the worker creating more value than what is needed to sustain their existence, which is essential for capital's survival (Marx, 1975a, p. 153). In Marxist fashion, surplus-value can be understood as closely related to the harsh realities of the proletariat's existence. Despite this connection, psychoanalysis suggests that the proletariat accepts the oppressive structure of surplus-value as a survival mechanism and a way to gain recognition as productive human asset of capitalism. This acceptance helps them manage the anxiety stemming from their disconnection from the world and enables them to cope with personal financial challenges such as debt and inflation. Therefore, this psychoanalytic perspective on Lacanian anxiety does not partake of the concept of surplus-enjoyment. Surplus-value is more associated with the anxiety and existential permanence of the proletariat, moving beyond the notion of surplus-enjoyment.

While surplus-value is often perceived negatively as a scenario of exploitation, Marx overlooks that it represents the proletariat's desire to maintain their value as labor. The proletariat actively chooses to become the barred subject ($) in order to exist within the framework of capitalism, which they see as the Other's *jouissance*. This choice reflects a perverse relationship with capitalism, where the proletariat submits to its demands to cope with anxiety and, in doing so, participates in the ongoing reproduction of capitalism as a form of realist ontology – an aspect of capitalist realism that Marx Fisher (2009), focused on collective mental illness (p. 73), tends to miss. Although capitalism assigns the proletariat to complete unproductive and wasteful jobs, it simultaneously serves as a means for them to fulfill their lack of desire, existence, and to cope with anxiety. Psychoanalytically speaking, the proletariat willingly embraces these roles, even when labeled by David Graber as "bullshit jobs", a point that Graber acknowledges as the activities that are not always necessarily that awful (Graber, 2018, p. 101). This dynamic reveals a desire for full recognition within capitalism, which complicates a one-dimensional view of class consciousness often associated with proletariat revolution. While the concept of "self-exploitation" could be advantageously noted as a form of self-motivation for both the middle class and the working class striving for success and to gain extreme self-respect in neoliberal capitalism (Han, 2015, p. 47), it does not sufficiently explore the psychoanalytic dimension of how self-exploitation reflects the proletariat's connection to the desire of the Other, as one of the problematical ways to deal with anxiety. For the proletariat, capitalism serves as a means for them to achieve existence while also psychoanalytically managing anxiety by themselves without the need for an actual clinical setting. However, the concept of self-exploitation overlooks the proletariat's efforts to ease the anxiety of feeling disconnected. The concept also fails to address the fundamental question of the proletariat's existence. In a psychoanalytic aspect, the proletariat comes to rely on capitalism to establish a clear sense of existence and to cope with anxiety, even though this reliance puts them at risk of engaging in a particular fantasy, preventing them from discovering their true desires.

A Psychoanalytic Act: *passage à l'acte*, acting-out, and a proletariat subject

In Seminar X, Lacan distinguishes between *passage à l'acte* and acting-out, placing a greater emphasis on the latter. He further develops the concept of acting-out from its initial stage to a more mature understanding in the unpublished Seminar XV, titled *The Psychoanalytic Act*. In the case of *passage à l'acte*, the subject experiences "the moment of the subject's greatest embarrassment" (Lacan, 2014j, p. 115). While the subject engaging in this action is historically grounded, they are unable to change any existing reality. Their only option is to "maintain themselves in their status as subject", ultimately feeling shame as they "rush and topple off the stage, out of the scene" (Lacan, 2014j, p. 115). In brief, the core structure of the subject's *passage à l'acte* involves "letting oneself drop", which highlights the subject's tragic experience of embarrassment, leading to a historical deadlock without any further progress (Lacan, 2014j, p. 115). In contrast, acting-out does not simply involve the subject "being dropped" and eventually exiting the scene. Instead, acting-out can be understood as "*letting oneself drop and getting back on stage*". The essence of acting-out arises from the failure to dominate the symbolic order – a form of "stupidity" – and transitions to a state of certainty. This marks a significant shift from being a subject defined by embarrassment, desperation, and failure to one driven by a principle that the subject faithfully believes in. This transition represents the core essence of certainty.

Departing from the traditional Marxist definition that narrowly defines the proletariat as a labor force whose surplus-value is extracted – specifically, those who exchange their investment of labor force for disproportionate wages – a psychoanalytic concept based on Lacan's distinction between *passage à l'acte* and acting-out emphasizes a particular characteristic of the proletariat subject. This psychoanalytical distinction presents two types of political subjects within what can be described as the theater of the proletariat.

First, there is the proletariat subject who embodies the act of taking action (*passage à l'acte*). Theoretically, they are historic subjects whose actions based on class consciousness and class struggle face significant social repercussions until they reach a breaking point – feeling depressed, stepping away from the spotlight, and ultimately choosing not to return. In reality, this type of proletariat may increasingly struggle to endure social repercussions and negative impacts affecting their lives. Consequently, some may opt to support a right-wing populist party that makes delusional promises to defend the interest of the proletariat: this is the greatest moment in the subject's embarrassment, as suggested by Lacan and noted earlier in the chapter. Others may abandon traditional Marxist views and instead align themselves with cultural wokeism, unless they find the best alternatives for themselves.

Second, there are the resilient and determined proletariat subjects who engage in action (Lacan's acting-out). Theoretically, they are not only historic subjects but also, amid inequality, setbacks, and violence, they transform their ignorance into certainty. They refuse to leave the stage and consistently return to it. In real life, this type of proletariat still upholds traditional Marxist principles. Despite experiencing pain and suffering, they remain committed to a Marxist stance, even when faced with various political options within the Left.

Acting-out and **objet a***: a proletariat subject, stupidity, and certainty*

In discussing the concept of certainty and the subject's inclination to connect with the *objet a* – a characteristic of the signifier of excess, the remainder, and the particular dimension of desire that lies outside the intelligibility of the Other – Lacan explores the notion of "acting-out". Acting-out illustrates the subject's speech act, which reveals not the truth but a façade – a mask – designed to conceal or veil something from the Other. However, this speech act does not hide the truth from the subject itself. Lacan states, "acting-out is essentially monstration, showing, which is doubtless veiled, but not veiled in and of itself" (Lacan, 2014j, p. 124). According to Lacan, acting-out is paradoxical, embodying a non-binary relationship between visibility and invisibility. Initially, visibility is captured through the subject's speech act, but this act serves as a trap: it is a mask that the subject dupes the Other. Upon closer examination, this speech act conceals something invisible – specifically, the truth about the subject, which is linked to the *objet a*, which remains hidden from the gaze of the Other. The essence of this invisibility is the *objet a* – a "remainder" or "offcut" that is lost in the relationship between subject and the Other (Lacan, 2014j, p. 124). In this sense, acting-out is directed toward the Other (Lacan, 2014j, p. 123), allowing the Other to remain unaware of the unknown desires that the subject harbors secretly. This ultimately leads to an invention of symptom in the domain of the Other, as Lacan suggests:

> *What is original about this acting-out and this demonstration of an unknown desire? The symptom is the same. Acting-out is a symptom. The symptom shows itself as something else too. The proof is that it has to be interpreted.*
> (Lacan, 2014j, p. 125 italics original)

The passage discusses the role of an analyst in a clinical setting, focusing on the interpretation of the analysand's hidden desires. During sessions, the analyst often encounters the transference of these unknown desires. It is the analyst's responsibility to recognize and interpret the *objet a*, ultimately revealing to the analysand the painful truth that such an imaginative object may not actually exist. Even if it does exist, it is unlikely to align with the analysand's expectations. The analyst faces two main choices: the first option is to assert authority by outright rejecting the analysand's unknown desires, labeling them as impossible. The second option, though disingenuous, allows the analysand's desires to persist by falsely suggesting that the *objet a* remains a viable possibility. However, a Lacanian psychoanalyst adopts a third approach. This third option involves conveying to the analysand that the *objet a* is symptomatically permissible. It serves as a signifier of desire; when the subject approaches or eventually possesses it, the expected desire linked to that object transforms into something else. According to the principle of dialectics, this indicates that even if the subject does attain the *objet a*, it often leads to disappointment, resulting in a sense of loss and nothingness rather than fulfillment. Lacan encapsulated this notion by stating,

> when you encounter it, you can be quite certain that it is an *a* for the subject. This creates a kind of connection that is widespread but can be difficult to manage because an a that is significant for the subject may become the most inconvenient superego.
>
> (Lacan, 2014j, p. 122)

Following Lacan, the principle of acting-out can shed light on the proletariat subject and the unknown desire – the *objet a* such as a communist world – in three probable outlooks regarding the proletariat subject and the *objet a*. Remarkably, the first two perspectives point out stupidity while the third one indicates certainty.

First, proletariat subjects have faced a prohibition of their *objet a*, particularly when it comes to achieving higher social justice, a fair redistribution of resources, social welfare, and significant reforms – capping off at the radical vision of a communist society. These unfulfilled desires can never be realized in reality because the current right-wing government, aligned with wealthy elites who benefit from tax avoidance and economic privilege, acts as a mechanism of repression, stifling these ambitions. Consequently, this results in the first form of Lacanian stupidity characteristic of the proletariat: they become marginalized, unable to impact the existing social dynamics, and find it difficult to regain their agency: the proletariat subject is dropped, unable to influence the symbolic social relationship, and never gets up again. It is possible that the subject of stupidity will find and seek another object of desire, which they expect to fulfill them, but that will not be possible.

Second, proletariat subjects have often been misled by the official narrative that blames immigrants for stealing jobs, creating social inequality. This narrative suggests that the root of their struggles lies in immigrants depriving them of opportunities, rather than addressing the deeper issues within the capitalist system itself. Psychoanalytically, the idea of reducing social inequality remains a potential goal – what is referred to as *objet a* – if the proletariat unifies and supports misguided decisions made by right-wing factions. However, this reliance on a narrative fabricated by the far-right ultimately leads to ignorance. It prevents the proletariat from recognizing the true causes of their situation. The real source of social inequality is capitalism, evidenced by the extraction of surplus-value from the labor of the proletariat. The government prioritizes subsidies for the wealthy and allocates funds to support national banks, all while neglecting social welfare for the poor. These actions reveal the true causes of social inequality, which should be addressed, rather than blaming immigrants.

Finally, the most significant idea emerging from Marxism is the belief that the proletariat must let themselves fall and then rise to the stage. As Marx (2007) states in "On Feuerbach" the proletariat needs to attain "perceptual materialism", a human society isolated from bourgeois society, which emphasizes the goal of establishing a communist society (p. 118). From a psychoanalytic perspective, the world beyond capitalism can be viewed as the *objet a*, representing both an excess and a signifier that exists outside the gaze of the Other – capitalism itself. However, as Lacan cautions, the *objet a* designates the enigmatic and unintelligible character of desire that disrupts the whole totalizing chain of symbolic meaning; once the subject attains it, it can symptomatically transform into something else. This suggests that if a communist world were to be realized, it might create a gap in desire and a feeling of unfulfillment for the proletariat, who may find it challenging to fully embrace and sustain this new reality; albeit with dissatisfaction. Therefore, what remains certain for the proletariat is that they must rise to the stage – acting-out – recognizing that the disharmony between themselves and the *objet a* called communism highlights the most inconvenient aspects of their superego.

The new saint? Degrowth communism, acting-out, and politics of certainty

What will the world look like after capitalism? Is there anyone – any Marxist – who dares to speak the truth or has the vision to imagine a future for everyone, especially for the proletariat? These questions are significant as they may fulfill Lacan's objective of finding a method and means to exit capitalism. This leads to another question: who will be the saint that saves everyone and liberates the proletariat from the constraints of capitalism?

In the past, there was a hypothesis concerning Lacanian scholars about exiting capitalism without needing a saint. However, the current academic landscape is evolving. It seems increasingly possible to exit capitalism by seeking a savior, or what could be considered a saint. This saint is neither a Lacanian Left nor a proponent of radical democracy, but Kohei Saito, a Japanese Marxist scholar whose impactful works display remarkable personal bravery in proposing solutions for the world's poly-crises. His two significant monographs, *Marx in the Anthropocene* (2020) and *Slow Down* (2024), are analytically rich and deserve thorough theoretical discussion. To some extent, Saito's concept of degrowth communism offers a guiding principle for the politics of the proletariat, aiming to envision a new society separable from capitalism.

Therefore, this section will first provide an analysis of Saito's characterization and conceptualization of degrowth communism, followed by a theoretical exploration of Lacanian psychoanalytic concepts – specifically anxiety, acting-out, and certainty – introducing an awareness of and some concerns regarding his ideas.

Kohei Saito's degrowth communism: proletariat, politics, and the fourth future

Degrowth communism is a concept derived from Marx's later vision of a different social framework that stands sharply in contrast to imperial capitalism. This idea integrates an analytical examination of political economy and ecology, along with Marx's reflections on pre-capitalist societies. Saito's analysis of Marx's works and his emphasis on the later writings, in particular, lead to the compelling conclusion that "Marx ultimately became a degrowth communist" (Saito, 2020, p. 173).

The idea of Marx as a degrowth communist thinker is valid, particularly when considering Saito's critical inquiry into the complete works of Marx and Engels, known as the *Marx-Engels-Gesamtausgabe* (*MEGA*). This analysis leads to a reinterpretation of Marx's overall thought process. The *MEGA* symbolizes Marx's ambition to reformulate a conception of history that goes beyond merely revising his historical materialism. It represents a substantial demonstration of Marx's vision for a radically different alternative society, specifically a degrowth communism. The "last Marx", or the Marx who advocates for degrowth communism, engages deeply with subjects such as natural science and the history of pre-capitalist societies, including agrarian communes in Russia and other non-Western societies in Asia, Africa, and Latin America. This intensive research empowers the last Marx to become an anti-Anthropocene thinker. His alternative vision for society seeks to save humanity from the destructive forces of capitalism, preventing us from heading toward negativity and ecological collapse on a global scale.

The concept of degrowth communism offers a fundamental metaphysical perspective on universal politics, emphasizing the collective efforts of subaltern people in both Western and non-Western countries to slow down economic growth. This movement seeks to eliminate the negative impacts that capitalism, characterized by anthropocentrism, has generated globally. Degrowth communism also advocates for industrialized or developed nations to adopt a different mode of economic metabolism quickly. It highlights a transition away from the current capitalist practices that accelerate the consumption of natural resources toward an alternative approach reminiscent of pre-capitalist societies, such as agrarian communes. These societies are often viewed as having greater awareness and rationality in managing human interaction with nature. This alternative knowledge represents a reawakening of consciousness that coincides with the revival of agrarian communes. It aims to guide society toward a steady-state economy, which can be described as "a stationary and circular economy without economic growth" (Saito, 2020, p. 207).

This vision reflects Marx's ideological objective of reviving the image of pre-capitalist societies, which pose a threat to the prevalence of global capitalism and its mode of production characterized by infinite capital accumulation. Degrowth communism represents a practice akin to a steady economy of pre-capitalist societies, regulating the use of land and natural resources. This approach contributes to the deceleration of economic growth while simultaneously preventing further degradation of ecological systems. This practice is also referred to as "communism in living" (Saito, 2020, p. 208). This concept envisions communism as a dynamic entity that represents a new mode of production, likely and probably defined by self-sufficiency. It also inspires an imagination for a new form of social production that serves as an alternative to the capitalist mode of production. This new economic practice aims to create an alternative mode of production that moves away from the pursuit of economic growth tied to endless capital accumulation.

In addition, Saito outlines a vision of degrowth communism that consists of five essential pillars (2024, pp. 194–204): (A) *transitioning to a use-value based economy* that emphasizes the end of mass production and consumption. (B) *shortening work hours* to allow workers to use their free time to produce necessary goods for society. This approach does not imply that degrowth communism will necessarily lead to a higher unemployment rate or less employment. (C) *abolishing the uniform division of labor*, which allows workers to autonomously choose creative work. To prevent routine tasks, workers would rotate jobs, enabling them to enhance their skills by engaging in various types of work. (D) *democratizing the production process* to contribute to economic deceleration while empowering workers to participate in democratic decisions regarding the means of production. In other words, workers would be allowed to decide democratically what, how, and how much should be produced (Saito,

2024, p. 202). This practice aims to move away from "the tyranny of capital", which represents swift, autocratic decision-making by capitalists. (E) *prioritizing essential work*, particularly "labor-intensive essential work", which refers to jobs that machinery cannot replace. Saito insists that "degrowth communism will transform our society into one that values these labor-intensive industries" (2024, p. 203). These roles are often perceived as high-cost and low-productivity sectors of the economy, such as care work.

Degrowth communism, as outlined by Saito, represents what he describes as the fourth future (Saito, 2024, p. 68). He identifies the first future as *climate fascism*, which reflects a societal ignorance where people continue to accelerate economic growth to uphold the status quo of capitalism (Saito, 2024, p. 69). The second future, termed *barbarism*, envisions a world descending into a "Hobbesian state of nature", characterized by a "war of all against all". In this scenario, individual interests and selfishness prevail above all else as climate change worsens. The third future, called *climate Maoism*, advocates for the promotion of the free market and liberal democracy yet relies on centralized state power to create and redistribute equality. However, it does not discard the same old approaches to combat climate change. Ultimately, Saito's preferred vision, the fourth future, is *degrowth communism*. This concept rejects both climate fascism and barbarism, as well as the state-centric approach of climate Maoism. In short, degrowth communism emphasizes the retrieval of Marx's research regarding (a) various types of pre-capitalist societies, (b) communism in living, and (c) the five pillars. It advocates for individuals to develop strategies to confront the climate crisis based on the principle of autonomy, aiming for "a just and sustainable future society" (Saito, 2024, p. 70).

A psychoanalytic reading of degrowth communism: Lacan, a second dimension of anxiety, acting-out, and certainty

This section connects Lacanian thought with degrowth communism, a process one can refer to as a psychoanalytic reading of degrowth communism. Although degrowth communism can be viewed as a foundational concept for the politics of the proletariat, Lacan's insights on anxiety, acting-out, and certainty offer a critical perspective for intellectual engagement with Saito's conceptualization. The arguments presented in this section will be organized into three main points.

First, Saito's concept of degrowth communism exemplifies a psychoanalytic act, while also suggesting that Saito himself may embody a Lacanian subject, generally known as the "divided subject". Lacan suggests that a psychoanalytic act revitalizes the process that produces sameness. He argues that such an act not only revokes the current state but also seeks to renew what was once considered the enlightened act (Lacan, 1967). According to Lacan, a psychoanalytic act results from the subject being affected by exploitation, and this capitalist influence on the subject precipitates the subject to perform an act that calls for revolution (Lacan, 1967). However, this does not mean that Lacan is a proponent of Marxism, and asserting that he aligns with a leftist ideology may not be entirely justified. Lacan also notes that after a revolution, there remains a significant challenge concerning the castration of the subject as a thinking being; this will certainly be a crisis as thinking in the communist order will be dominated by the intelligentsia (Lacan, 1967). This phallic dominance is seen as inevitable in a communist order. Therefore, the Lacanian psychoanalytic Act does not simply surrender to oppression; it seeks to sublimate oppression into a revolution. Yet, it raises skepticism about the revolution, particularly regarding the potential negative consequences, such as the evaporation of Man as a thinking being within the communist world.

Nonetheless, degrowth communism can be understood as a psychoanalytic Act as it attempts to break free from the repetitive compulsion of capitalist actions that lead to historical sameness and ultimately threaten global extinction. Given the five pillars previously mentioned, it is unjust to label degrowth communism as a movement against progress. Instead, this movement has the potential to negate the repetitive actions of capitalism that falsely claim to embody enlightenment. Degrowth communism represents a materialist interpretation of Lacan's psychoanalytic act by opposing three competitive futures: climate fascism, barbarism, and climate Maoism, all of which are entrenched in the capitalist symbolic order. This aligns with Lacan's emphasis on the psychoanalytic act as revealing a path toward ontological difference.

Is it possible for Lacanian theory to reposition degrowth communism within a clinical setting, where the relationship between the psychoanalyst and the analysand is central? If this is feasible, then through a lens of degrowth communism, Saito, as a subject, may reflect what Lacan refers to as the divided subject. This concept addresses the subject as being ontologically folded with two conflicting forms of thinking and self-reflection regarding both the self and others, resembling a dialectical subject. The first aspect of this divided subject is the psychoanalyst, who operates from the master discourse. In this scenario, Saito occupies the position of the Hegelian master. His desire to wake others to mutually save and change the world helps position him as a discourse of the master: a saint. Degrowth communism acts as the master discourse that shapes the collective consciousness of the proletariat, urging them to recognize the oppressive nature of capitalism, its Anthropocene consequences, and the deterioration of the ecological system. The proletariat, awakened from the false consciousness imposed by capitalism, can be understood psychoanalytically as the analysand – a patient receiving treatment from Saito, who assumes a Hegelian position of the master discourse.

The second aspect of the divided subject portrays Saito as the analysand or the hysterical subject. In this role, a hysterical subject projects a hidden desire onto the psychoanalyst, who must avoid succumbing to countertransference. In this aspect, the psychoanalyst here is not a Hegelian master but rather a Zen master.

A metaphor of the psychoanalyst as a Zen master is essential to the analyst's discourse. This is why the first sentence on the first page of Lacan's first seminar begins with his mention of a Buddhist master:

> The master breaks the silence with anything – with a sarcastic remark, with a kick-start. This is how a Buddhist master conducts his search for meaning, according to the technique of Zen. It behoves the students to find out for themselves the answer to their own questions. The master does not teach *ex cathedra* a ready made science; he supplies an answer when the students are on the verge of finding it.
>
> (Lacan, 1991, p. 1: italics originals)

While in the first aspect, Saito is assumed as the Hegelian master, the Zen master refers to anyone who listens carefully to the subject's desire to speak, their wants, and aspirations, without reacting in a counterproductive way. The Zen master needs to regard the subject's thoughts, affects, and transference as objects of desire. Lacan instructs that "the operation of the psychoanalytic act ought to reduce this subject [the analysand] to the *objet a*" (Lacan, 1967). Thus, endowed with his understanding of degrowth communism, and psychoanalytically speaking, the notion reveals Saito as a hysterical subject who transfers his thoughts on degrowth communism to anyone willing to listen carefully to his unconscious desires as well as his vision for a world beyond capitalism.

Ultimately, reading from a psychoanalytical perspective, Saito's exploration of degrowth communism illustrates that he embodies a Lacanian divided subject. On the one hand, he is seen as a psychoanalyst emerging from the Hegelian position of the master discourse; on the other hand, he can be regarded as the analysand or a hysterical subject actively transmitting his *objet a* to a psychoanalyst – anyone – through Saito's free association.

Degrowth communism can be understood as an *objet a*. Its foundation lies in the principle of universal politics and its promotion of a type of pre-capitalist society, which generates desires that extend beyond the boundaries of symbolic capitalism. Degrowth communism is the Real as it embodies an excess that has not yet been integrated into the symbolic order. Degrowth communism reflects what Freud refers to as "*niderfallen*" – an object that, the closer the subject gets to it, the more it tends to provoke anxiety. This aligns with the second dimension of anxiety mentioned earlier. In other words, in the context of historical materialism and capitalism, degrowth communism can be viewed as the excess and the irreducible remainder that exists outside of capitalism, functioning as Lacanian *objet a*. However, as long as the relationship between the subject and the *objet a* remains one where the *objet a* forms an enigmatic non-relationship to the subject's pursuit of desire – an idea suggested by Lacan regarding *objet a* – it can lead to frustration and may ultimately be counterproductive. Degrowth communism embodies Saito's pursuit of truth and engages with a master-signifier concerning the future of humanity. Nonetheless, degrowth communism may encounter obstacles – referred to as the cutting effect of the Real – that could create gaps or disruptions in this signifier. Ultimately, this approach may reveal a shocking meaning that differentiates itself from its original interpretation as articulated by Saito.

Then, to kill off anxiety in the second dimension, it is posited with optimism that degrowth communism would not incline toward what Lacan calls the object "that which deceives not" and will not produce and lead to the "subject as real" or the subject finally homed with *objet a* but finds it unable to fulfill a whole satisfaction, as noted earlier. Ultimately, it is also hoped that degrowth communism will not share the same quality of Hegel's "a glove turned inside out", in which the object is the object present at hand, but resisting the hand of the subject until the subject is pressurized to live in pursuit of capitalism – a sameness of Being – without true historical reversion. In short, degrowth communism is expected to overcome Lacan's caution that for the *objet a*, "its ultimate mainspring may elude him indefinitely", as mentioned earlier.

Third, it is important to note that Saito's work is gaining increasing attention from both international academics and individuals outside of academia. From a Lacanian perspective, degrowth communism should not be equated with Lacan's concepts of stupidity and *passage à l'acte* but rather with the ideas of acting-out and certainty. To clarify, Lacan's notion of stupidity refers to the profound disconnection that follows an initial connection between the subject and the *objet a*, which leads to the subject's re-experience of lack. Stupidity highlights the subject's *passage à l'acte*, at risk resulting in the subject's absolute fall, and the subject looks for a new object of desire that wholly satisfies them. It is unfair to suggest that Saito's proposal of degrowth communism embodies Lacan's concept of stupidity. Because it cannot be asserted that degrowth communism will necessarily lead everyone to experience loss repeatedly. Additionally, characterizing Saito as someone who doubts himself is a significant misrepresentation. Similarly, it is not accurate to argue that degrowth communism represents a form of surrender; Saito consistently posits degrowth communism as the foundational "fourth future", as previously noted.

Ultimately, it is more justifiable to view degrowth communism in relation to Lacan's concepts of acting-out and certainty. To clarify again, the relationship between acting-out and certainty highlights the signifier of a subject who is "letting oneself drop and getting up on the stage" (Lacan, 2014j, p. 114), and who dares to embrace dissatisfaction emanated from the object of desire. From a psychoanalytic perspective, it is theoretically possible to connect anxiety to degrowth communism. If degrowth communism ultimately materializes similarly to Lacan's metaphor of "a closed book on the subject", it may represent an object that promises complete satisfaction but instead results in a certain level of dissatisfaction and unfulfillment for the subject. As suggested by Jenny Edkins, certainty can be viewed dialectically as the will and a continuity to act, which creates uncertainty – something that is unmeasurable and potentially disruptive – at the core of all present things (Edkins, 2019, pp. 5–9). As a result, the subject will likely experience anxiety as degrowth communism unfolds, even briefly. If this scenario were to occur in the future, it is anticipated that Saito and his degrowth communism members would metaphorically "get up on the stage", as it is through this immediate action called a drive for the subject's acting-out after the near Absolute Fall that they could potentially liberate themselves from anxiety.

In summary, there exists a theoretical connection between Marx and Lacan, suggesting that Marx's concept of the proletariat is linked to the notion of surplus-value, which in turn reflects what Lacan refers to as the surplus-enjoyment of the capitalist subject. However, this chapter proposes an alternative perspective: surplus-value also highlights the relationship between the proletariat and anxiety in two ways. First, the proletariat often conforms to the capitalist demand for productivity as a means to manage financial burdens and alleviate anxiety stemming from social isolation. Second, while anxiety can serve as a signal of resistance to capitalism, visions of a world beyond capitalism – such as communism – can lead to disappointment and disillusionment due to the unrealistic expectations surrounding them. From a psychoanalytic standpoint, the proletariat's psychoanalytic Act can manifest in two forms: as a *passage à l'acte*, which indicates a failure to navigate social complexities while looking for a new thing instead of the old, culminating in the subject of stupidity, or as *acting-out*, which reflects a commitment to their desires in the face of pain and dissatisfaction, reflecting the emergence of the subject of certainty.

Reference list

Edkins, J. (2019). *Change and the Politics of Certainty*. Manchester: Manchester University Press.

Fisher, M. (2009). *Capitalist Realism: Is There No Alternative?*. Hants: O Books.

Graber, D. (2018). *Bullshit Jobs: A Theory*. New York: Simon & Schuster Books.

Han, B-C. (2015). *The Burnout Society*. Translated by Erik Butler. Stanford: Stanford University Press.

Lacan, J. (1967). Unpublished Text. *The Seminar of Jacques Lacan Book XV: The Psychoanalytical Act*. English translation is from an unpublished text by Cormac Gallagher. Available at: https://www.lacaninireland.com/wp-content/uploads/2010/06/Book-15-The-Psychoanalytical-Act.pdf. Accessed: May 14, 2025.

Lacan, J. (1991). 'Overture to the Seminar', in *The Seminar of Jacques Lacan Book I: Freud's Papers on Technique*. Translated by John Forrester. Edited by Jacques-Alain Miller. London and New York: W.W. Norton & Company.

Lacan, J. (2006). 'The Subversion of the Subject and the Dialectic of Desire in the Freudian Unconscious', in *Écrits: The First Complete Edition in English*. Translated by Bruce Fink. London and New York: W.W. Norton & Company.

Lacan, J. (2014a). 'Anxiety in the Net of Signifiers', in *The Seminar of Jacques Lacan Book X: Anxiety*. Edited by Jacques Alain-Miller. Translated by A. R. Price. Cambridge and Malford: Polity Press.

Lacan, J. (2014b). 'Anxiety, Sign of Desire', in *The Seminar of Jacques Lacan Book X: Anxiety*. Edited by Jacques Alain-Miller. Translated by A. R. Price. Cambridge and Malford: Polity Press.

Lacan, J. (2014c). 'Anxiety, Signal of the Real', in *The Seminar of Jacques Lacan Book X: Anxiety*. Edited by Jacques Alain-Miller. Translated by A. R. Price. Cambridge and Malford: Polity Press.

Lacan, J. (2014d). 'Aphorisms on Love', in *The Seminar of Jacques Lacan Book X: Anxiety*. Edited by Jacques Alain-Miller. Translated by A. R. Price. Cambridge and Malford: Polity Press.

Lacan, J. (2014e). 'Beyond Castration Anxiety', in *The Seminar of Jacques Lacan Book X: Anxiety*. Edited by Jacques Alain-Miller. Translated by A. R. Price. Cambridge and Malford: Polity Press.

Lacan, J. (2014f). 'From the *a* to the Names-of-the-Father', in *The Seminar of Jacques Lacan Book X: Anxiety*. Edited by Jacques Alain-Miller. Translated by A. R. Price. Cambridge and Malford: Polity Press.

Lacan, J. (2014g). 'From the Cosmos to the *Unheimliche*', in *The Seminar of Jacques Lacan Book X: Anxiety*. Edited by Jacques Alain-Miller. Translated by A. R. Price. Cambridge and Malford: Polity Press.

Lacan, J. (2014h). 'Not Without Having It', in *The Seminar of Jacques Lacan Book X: Anxiety*. Edited by Jacques Alain-Miller. Translated by A. R. Price. Cambridge and Malford: Polity Press.

Lacan, J. (2014i). 'On a Circle That Is Irreducible to a Point', in *The Seminar of Jacques Lacan Book X: Anxiety*. Edited by Jacques Alain-Miller. Translated by A. R. Price. Cambridge and Malford: Polity Press.

Lacan, J. (2014j). '*Passage à l'acte* and Acting-Out', in *The Seminar of Jacques Lacan Book X: Anxiety*. Edited by Jacques Alain-Miller. Translated by A. R. Price. Cambridge and Malford: Polity Press.

Lacan, J. (2014k). 'That Which Deceives Not', in *The Seminar of Jacques Lacan Book X: Anxiety*. Edited by Jacques Alain-Miller. Translated by A. R. Price. Cambridge and Malford: Polity Press.

Lacan, J. (2014l). 'That Which Deceives', in *The Seminar of Jacques Lacan Book X: Anxiety*. Edited by Jacques Alain-Miller. Translated by A. R. Price. Cambridge and Malford: Polity Press.

Lacan, J. (2014m). 'The Cause of Desire', in *The Seminar of Jacques Lacan Book X: Anxiety*. Edited by Jacques Alain-Miller. Translated by A. R. Price. Cambridge and Malford: Polity Press.

Lacan, J. (2021). 'Introduction', in *The Seminar of Jacques Lacan Book IV: The Object Relation*. Edited by Jacques Alain-Miller. Translated by A. R. Price. Cambridge and Malford: Polity Press.

Marx, K. (1975a). *Theories of Surplus-Value Part I*. Edited by S. Ryazanskaya. Translated by Emile Burns. Moscow: Progress Publishers.

Marx, K. (1975b). *Theories of Surplus-Value Part II*. Edited by S. Ryazanskaya. Translated by Emile Burns. Moscow: Progress Publishers.

Marx, K. (1975c). *Theories of Surplus-Value Part III*. Edited by S. Ryazanskaya. Translated by Emile Burns. Moscow: Progress Publishers.

Marx, K. (2007). "On Feuerbach", in *Marx Early Political Writings*. Edited and Translated by Joseph O'Malley in collaboration with Richard A. Davis. Cambridge: Cambridge University Press.

Saito, K. (2020). *Marx in the Anthropocene: Towards the Idea of Degrowth Communism*. Cambridge: Cambridge University Press.

Saito, K. (2024). *Slow Down: How Degrowth Communism Can Save The Earth*. Translated by Brain Bergstrom. London: Weidenfeld & Nicolson.

7 Trauma as a political factor

Rethinking dialectical materialism and the proletariat as post-traumatic subject

This chapter emphasizes Jacques Lacan's concepts of the RSI and how they contribute to Lacan's theory of trauma, particularly Imaginary-Trauma, Symbolic-Trauma, and Real-Trauma. It is Real-Trauma that gives rise to the notion of capitalist trauma, acknowledging its prominent role as a political factor for the proletariat. This framework suggests that capitalist trauma reveals a symptomatic connection among presentism, materialism, and universalism. In contrast to an affirmative Lacanian-Žižekian political account – where enjoyment is a political factor – this chapter considers trauma itself as a crucial political element. The concept of capitalist trauma prompts a reevaluation of Karl Marx's dialectical materialism, exploring both the alignment and tension between capitalist trauma and dialectical materialism. Additionally, this chapter proposes the idea of the proletariat subject as a post-traumatic subject – one whose way of life actively challenges the existing order while embracing inherent dangers – this perspective on subjectivity is omitted from Marx's consideration of the proletariat. Ultimately, it aims to engage in theoretical and epistemic dialogues with postcolonialism and Laclauian politics by connecting the concept of capitalist trauma with the post-traumatic character of the proletariat.

Like other previous chapters, this chapter is structured according to the four fundamental dimensions of the proletariat discourse: psyche, existence, subject, and politics. The first section develops a Lacanian theory of trauma as a dialectic of the psyche involving three interconnected knots related to the proletariat. Imaginary-Trauma involves the self-imaginary of the proletariat, highlighting issues like post-traumatic stress disorder (PTSD) from workplace bullying, which depoliticizes their struggle against capitalism and erodes trust and solidarity necessary for workplace democratization. Symbolic-Trauma centers on identity and postcolonial politics, leading the proletariat to focus on identity differences (e.g., race and gender) instead of revolutionary politics, which ultimately distracts from confronting capitalist trauma as a universalism. Real-Trauma, the most significant, this trauma emphasizes that capitalist issues are present realities – a multiple crisis affecting all subjects. But recognizing Real-Trauma can lead

DOI: 10.4324/9781003657781-7

individuals back to Imaginary or Symbolic-Traumas, complicating revolutionary efforts. The triad of trauma – Real-Trauma, Imaginary-Trauma, and Symbolic-Trauma – affects the proletariat's psyche. According to the principles of dialectic, this means that those proletariats who experience capitalist trauma as Real-Trauma understand that they must oppose capitalism, yet they may not succeed in the act of revolution. Instead, a psyche of their own will urge them to regress into Imaginary-Trauma (feeling that solidarity is unattainable) and Symbolic-Trauma (viewing proletariat politics merely as identity politics), complicating the path to revolutionary action. This interplay creates a challenging mental struggle for the proletariat, who endures this dialectical psychical condition. If the proletariat is thought to have this dialectical psychological condition, it is unjust for traditional Marxism to simplify the natural complexities of the proletariat's psyche to mere class consciousness.

The second section examines capitalist trauma through the lens of dialectical materialism. It argues that Marx and Engels' dialectical materialism, which critiques capitalism as a material condition, shares a commonality with the concept of Real-Trauma. However, it also suggests that dialectical materialism contains elements of a communist fantasy. The idea of "from each according to his abilities, to each according to his needs", where "labor has become not merely a means to live but the foremost need in life" (Marx, 2021b, pp. 214–215), can conflict with the notion of Lacanian enjoyment, where desire thrives on the experience of lack. In a capitalist framework, this lack fuels an insatiable pursuit of fulfillment. However, in communism, the proposed new mode of production and its associated social structure could diminish enjoyment by transforming it from a state of excess into one of necessity, ability, and need. This shift might lead to a society focused on living within strict necessities, with less enjoyment, where the proletariat in the new world is related to what is only needed in life.

The third section proposes the idea of the proletariat as a post-traumatic subject. Rather than viewing the proletariat merely as a labor force exploited for capitalist gain, this notion, grounded in Lacanian trauma theory, highlights a more complex understanding of proletariat subjectivity. While Marx aims to position the proletariat as a key political agency in emancipatory politics, he overlooks the importance of psychoanalytic subjectivity. This perspective suggests that the proletariat must actively detach itself from the symbolic realm – essentially, the structures of capitalism – to confront the inherent dangers it faces. The post-traumatic subject may embody the proletariat's experience of Real-Trauma, a trauma linked to capitalism itself, and likely possesses a motivation to oppose capitalist systems. However, this subjectivity is not monolithic; it can fluctuate and may be disrupted by Imaginary-Trauma and Symbolic-Trauma. Such disruptions can create internal tensions and divisions within the proletariat's formation of the subject, and this can recede proletariat as a subject of resistance. This concept aligns with the idea of a split subject, as advanced by Lacanian psychoanalysis, which seeks to explore the nature of subjectivity and uncover its underlying truths. Marx and traditional Marxism should reflect on whether they wish to understand the proletariat as a complex entity or merely use its subjectivity for ideological purposes. Acknowledging the proletariat as a multifaceted and fragmented subject brings everyone closer to understanding its true nature, rather than reducing it for ideological purposes.

Finally, the fourth section will expand on the ideas of capitalist trauma and the proletariat as a post-traumatic subject to foster critical discussions with postcolonial politics and identity politics. It argues that a universal approach to emancipatory politics cannot neglect a critique of capitalism. Nevertheless, it is worth noting that efforts to combat capitalism, relying on the proletariat as a subject of resistance, face challenges due to the complexities of proletariat subjectivity and the dialectical reflections that arise within it.

A Lacanian theory of trauma: A dialectic of the psyche

Imaginary-Trauma: depoliticization and the Hegelian master and slave

In the diagram (see Figure 7.1), the Imaginary highlights the "I" (*je*) striving to achieve unity of the self (Lacan, 1999a, p. 90). A critical aspect of this process is Lacan's assertion that the formation of the "I" cannot attain a sense of unity without depending on the linguistic stage, specifically the realm of the Other. Therefore, the Imaginary represents a psychological stage characterized by a tension between individuals, language, and the Other. One example of the

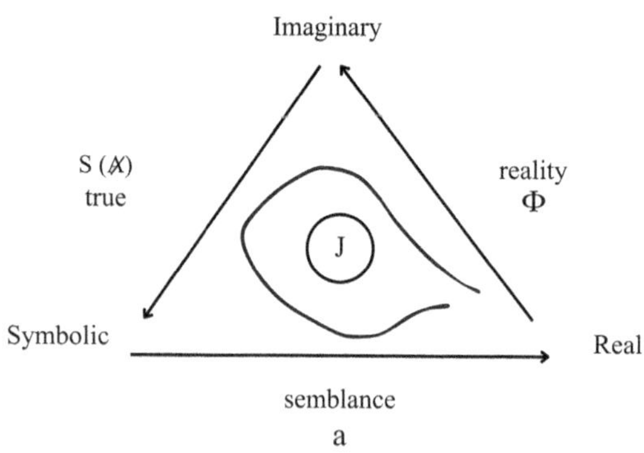

Figure 7.1 Relation between objects and Lacanian triad RSI (Real, Symbolic, and Imaginary).

Source: Figure adapted from Lacan, J. (1999). *The Seminar of Jacques Lacan Book XX: On Feminine Sexuality*. Edited by Jacques-Alain Miller. Translated by Bruce Fink. London and New York: W.W. Norton Company. p. 90.

Imaginary is the mirror stage, which illustrates a child beginning to recognize their own reflection in a mirror. This recognition contrasts with the Other, serving as a foundation for understanding the self. The mirror stage is significant to the Imaginary because it marks the initial and rudimentary form of the subject, providing a primary stage for understanding the self in relation to the influence of the Other (*Autre*), represented as "A" in the diagram. This relationship aligns with the role of the Hegelian Master and its socio-linguistic influence in shaping the ego of the "I" (Lacan, 1999a, p. 90).

However, the ego docs not represent the true subject. Instead, it signifies a misidentification of the self. From Lacan's perspective, the ego is formed through the subject's social connection with the desire of the Other. Within this framework, the ego can be problematic; it often leads individuals to perceive things inaccurately. However, it remains essential for a sense of self and the ability to relate to other individuals. The imaginary aspect of the ego begins to take shape, yet it is not where the subject finds its true home. For the subject to reach this realization, self-interrogation is necessary to challenge the entire process surrounding it. In Lacan's graph, S (the barred A) represents not only the barred subject ($) but also the status of the ego. This status relates to the Other – the realm of language – that can cause misleading effects on the subject, leading them to lose their true sense of self and ultimately fail to find their home. There exists a tension between the Other – such as a psychoanalyst, who can be viewed as a Hegelian master – and the barred subject ($). This dynamic can be understood through Hegelian concepts of "the master's desire and the slave" (Lacan, 1981a, p. 254). The master often seeks to impose their will on the slave or barred subject, effectively depriving them of freedom and life, reducing them to a state of impure prestige. This situation reflects a lack of truth concerning the slave's true desire (Lacan, 1981c, p. 219).

Lacan's concept of the Imaginary allows for an exploration of the idea of Imaginary-Trauma. This notion suggests that a subject carries a scar from painful traumatic memories. The traumatized individual forms their ego based on these memories by distinguishing themselves from those who have not experienced such trauma. Consequently, trauma becomes a crucial psychoanalytical factor in the formation of the ego, helping the individual differentiate their painful experiences from those of others who remain unscathed by such intense suffering. Moreover, Imaginary-Trauma illustrates how a subject's ego formation relies on trauma, which facilitates the dominance of medical knowledge – akin to a Hegelian master – seeking to "rescue" the subject. A clear example of this is PTSD, which is commonly associated with traumatic experiences. Additionally, other forms of mental illness related to capitalism, such as workplace PTSD, manifest in various ways, including hypervigilance and difficulty concentrating, which can insidiously affect work performance (Peck, Drebing, and Schutt, 2002, p. 223). Workplace PTSD is a form of mental illness that significantly affects many proletariats. This reality excludes them from participating in the process of democratizing workplaces and fosters distrust in the system that prevents every worker from engaging in proper decision-making about the direction of the organization.

Imaginary-Trauma tends to also prioritize medical knowledge, which creates a scenario reminiscent of a Hegelian master-slave relationship. This emphasis can leave individuals politically uninformed and disengaged. To address PTSD, individuals often find themselves compelled to adhere to a mental health discourse that aligns with a medical framework, one that stigmatizes those dealing with trauma – such as patients suffering from workplace PTSD – as mere objects of medical intervention. By neglecting the idea that capitalism may be a root cause of such mental illnesses, individuals may view themselves solely as patients, missing the potential for self-realization akin to a Hegelian slave's revolution: it is a Hegelian master that underscores the suppression of the truth about the slave. This suppression occurs because the master imposes their desires onto the slave, causing the latter to become indistinguishably aligned with the master's identity. As a result, the slave's own desires and sense of self become entrapped in a complex mirroring process, the stage which is led by the master until the slave's desire is deprived of self-expression and dialectical reflection.

In short, Imaginary-Trauma is unfortunately politically inactive. It represents an overarching power that exerts control and produces knowledge through clinical practices aimed at curing mental illness. This discourse reflects a Hegelian master narrative that exerts medical power over traumatized individuals, simultaneously undermining the potential for a Hegelian slave revolution within the proletariat.

Symbolic-Trauma: postcolonialism, identity politics, and the absence of the universality of trauma

The symbolic order functions as both a structural framework that represents the role of law and order and as the realm of language, which plays a crucial role in an individual's construction of self. It embodies a construction of objective fantasy that connects with a subjective engagement and production of one's own fantasy. Psychoanalysis suggests that a person engages with language from the moment of birth, being immersed in it even before birth. For an individual to exist, they must be constituted, internalized, and mutually shaped by the demands of language. Lacan describes the transition from the disorientation of a pre-linguistic stage to the emergence of the subject within the symbolic order as the "anchoring point" (*point de capiton*), explaining it as "the signifier stops the otherwise infinite sliding of signification" (Lacan, 2006b, p. 681).

The concept of an anchoring point is notably different from that of a master-signifier, a distinction that Laclau often overlooks (Laclau, 2001, p. xi). An anchoring point refers to the process through which an individual is required to shape their subjectivity based on that anchoring point itself, forming the foundation, serving as a ground, for such a development. This process illustrates how the subject appears to establish a smooth and homogeneous relationship with the social order by learning to recognize the differences and similarities among the signs and signifiers prevalent in society. If this connection is misaligned, it can disrupt the subject's adherence to the Symbolic, potentially leading to the subject being perceived as delusional or abnormal by others. In contrast, a master-signifier arises from a subject's active engagement and production within the Symbolic and is linked to social dynamics and meaningful interactions, such as the act of asserting oneself as a sign in the field of discursivity in the pursuit of liberty, solidarity, and equality against oppressive regimes (Laclau, 2001, p. 112). Lacan suggests that there is no single, definitive master-signifier; meanings can change, and one discourse may refer to another. This means that what might be perceived as a master can also assume the role of a hysteric, and vice versa (Lacan, 1999b, p. 16). This idea poses challenges for individuals attempting to position themselves as a master-signifier, which can lead to feelings of ontological inconsistency. In contrast, Laclau often associates the anchoring point with the master-signifier and tends to depict political subjects as if they embody this concept. However, this perspective may overlook the complexities and internal struggles that these subjects experience. In other words, the fundamental difference between anchoring points and master-signifiers underscores the complexities of subjectivity and the challenges involved in establishing new social orders that require dialectical reflection.

Figure 7.1 illustrates how the subject eventually emerges as a divided entity, gradually shedding its resemblance to the Symbolic order. Specifically, it shows that when the subject transcends its superficial likeness – referred to as the subject for the Symbolic – it spontaneously attains the status of *objet a* (Lacan, 1999a, p. 90). In this context, the excess and surplus inherent in the subject struggle to coexist harmoniously with the Symbolic order's inability to access the darker aspects of the subject. A key characteristic of the *objet a* is its capacity to interrogate the Symbolic order or showing its actuality that exceeds societal norms that aim to enforce conformity. This Symbolic anchoring point does not serve as an end in itself but instead represents a departure for the subject. As long as the subject positions itself as the master-signifier, which will eventually fail, it merely represents an excess, a disparity, or surplus-enjoyment in relation to the divided subject. Without the potential for genuine social change, the divided subject can only question and dismantle the established symbolic framework. This divided subject is merely capable of questioning and dismantling the established symbolic framework, which itself is experiencing an ontological disparity. In short, both psychoanalytic concepts – the anchoring point characterized as ontological disparity and the master-signifier as an absolute failure – are recognized among typical Lacanians as having inherent and significant flaws from the outset, making them unsuitable components for any political theories such as radical democracy.

Lacan's concept of the Symbolic allows for the development of the idea of Symbolic-Trauma. Symbolic Trauma refers to the way individuals assert themselves as master-signifiers in response to an established Symbolic anchoring point. This concept involves the active symbolization of trauma as realized by the individual. The act of writing serves as an exemplification of Symbolic Trauma, asserting themselves as the master-signifier: an excess, a disparity, and the split subject. For survivors who have experienced and endured horrific incidents, their trauma is often conveyed through narratives in memoirs or as witnesses in legal proceedings. These trauma narratives can be seen as counterproductive to the hegemonic official narratives, an anchoring point presented by the government. This often leads to a demarcation in favor of identity formation – identity politics – and can foster social structural tribalism between groups of official governments assumed as perpetrators and the subaltern assumed as victims. In other words, the Manichean logic inherent in Symbolic-Trauma not only gives rise to collective trauma but also generates a sense of tribalism. This tribalism is violently desired by identity politics, especially in the current context of cultural wokeism. Wokeism focuses obsessively on anti-racial prejudice and anti-sexual discrimination. It praises a matter of socially constructed identity as emancipatory politics. However, it fails to address the capitalist trauma that universally causes negativities to all people, regardless of race, gender, and nationalities. It is not unexpected that Symbolic-Trauma, particularly the concept of the master-signifier, can support postcolonialism rather than lead to emancipation from capitalism. This concept allows subaltern cultures to express their identities within a linguistic framework that is free from imperial domination.

Postcolonialism's representation of traumatic memory serves the interests of proletariat politics as identity politics. If the government's narrative on trauma is considered the official version – acting as an anchoring point for every subject – then the postcolonial narrative is permitted to represent what Lacanian psychoanalysis designates as *object a*: a form of trauma that splits, transcends, and exceeds the government's portrayal, which seeks to uphold political order and nationalism. A postcolonial interpretation of symbolic trauma tends to narrate trauma in a way that risks distracting the proletariat from engaging in meaningful emancipatory politics. Instead, it may lead them to focus solely on the aspects of postcolonialism and identity politics. This includes the varied experiences of different groups within the proletariat, such as the white dominant and privileged proletariat, black proletariat, Asian proletariat, as well as male, female, and LGBTQ+ proletariat. It is worth considering this matter with a dialectical reflection. First, if the narration of trauma within postcolonialism is assumed to be a master-signifier, it is likely to collapse and ultimately fail. According to Lacan (2006a), "the narration, in fact, doubles the drama with a commentary without which no *mise-en-scène* would be possible" (p. 7). This indicates that when postcolonialism and identity politics emphasize their trauma narratives as primary symbols, these woke individuals may risk exaggerating the significance of their own identities in relation to social suppression, discrimination, and oppression. While there is some truth to this perspective, it ultimately fails to reveal the complete reality. This is because *mise-en-scène* is not equivalent to truth; instead, it creates an excess of truth until the truth itself is sanctified. Consequently, the postcolonial version of the Symbolic-Trauma generates a *mise-en-scène* that is certainly not the truth itself. Second, while Symbolic-Trauma can be beneficial for non-white proletariats who insist on narrating their experiences and for the resurgence of their postcolonial identity in contrast to the white proletariats, it is insufficient to elevate trauma to a universal level. Universal trauma connects an individual's consciousness to Real-Trauma, which includes capitalist trauma – an idea that will be addressed in the next section.

The Real-Trauma: the emergence of capitalist trauma as presentism, materialism, and universalism

In the diagram (Figure 7.1), the concept of the true precedes the Real. The true refers to the barred Other, which is not the truth itself but rather a mechanism that constructs the truth, creating a semblance of reality. The true is distinct from the Real, indicating that the Real has not yet been revealed. Lacan's well-known definition of the Real has been recognized since 1950. In Lacan's Seminar I, it is stated that the Real "is what resists symbolization absolutely" (Lacan, 1991, p. 66). To the right of the graph, there is an algebra of the empty set, Ø, which signifies the void and represents the existence of something that negates the fabricated truth (Lacan, 1999a, p. 90). This is the position of the Real, which exerts a cutting effect against the fabricated truth – the reality. In addition to the empty set, the Real functions together with Lacan's concept of *objet a*. In relation to *objet a*, the Real has two functions: first, it appears as a paradoxical absent presence, and second, it performs a cutting effect against the fabricated truth, thereby dismantling reality to some extent. Together, these functions encourage us to reconsider and reconstitute reality as an impossible wholeness.

Lacan's concept of the Real provides a framework for understanding what is termed Real-Trauma. Real-Trauma refers to a traumatic experience that individuals inevitably confront in the present. Real-Trauma encompasses individuals and their drastic actions, leading to a sense of emptiness – a void – where they feel unable to overcome their current circumstances. This dimension of trauma suggests that people do not want to die in vain; they actively try hard to challenge it but ultimately remain stuck, finding themselves fixated in the same place. In contrast to Derridean logic, which highlights trauma as the haunting image of the future and suggests that subjects risk being passively overtaken, consumed, and devoured by this image (Derrida, 1994, pp. 1–10) – a concept rooted in hauntology – Real-Trauma shifts the focus to the overwhelming present that shapes people's lives after their long-enduring attempts and endeavors to challenge the existing repressive circumstance. In short, Real-Trauma is the present moment that haunts the subject, rather than the ghosts of the past or specter of the future. Nonetheless, the term "Real-Trauma" encompasses three key elements: presentism, materialism, and universalism. These three elements are developed from the earlier representation of Real-Trauma, which presents a traumatized subject breaking through the official Symbolic narration of trauma (Supachalasai, 2017).

In terms of presentism, the concept of Real-Trauma requires a temporal dimension. It does not simply refer to a haunting memory of past trauma that afflicts the survivor of a life-threatening event. Instead, Real-Trauma is situated in the present context. It represents a situation where many individuals protest against their circumstances, yet this defiance often results in absolute failure, leaving them feeling trapped with no way out. Thus, Real-Trauma embodies a quality of presentism; it is not just a lingering effect of an unforgettable past memory that disturbs the individual. A fitting metaphor for Real-Trauma is a labyrinth. When individuals reach what they believe is the exit of the labyrinth – finding freedom and independence – they discover it leads back into another pathway within the labyrinth itself. For these individuals, this realization becomes a traumatic experience.

It is important to consider whether Real-Trauma represents idealism or materialism. For the purposes of this discussion, Real-Trauma is not idealism. The pain associated with it is tied to the current living conditions of individuals, rather than being an abstract suffering. Therefore, Real-Trauma embodies a material condition – one that signifies the concrete existence in which every individual is compelled to participate. Real-Trauma, thus, possesses a materialistic quality, reflecting the actual reality that shapes a subject's living situation. There are numerous individuals from various countries who protest against their precarious conditions. However, they often find that the circumstances are insurmountable. For some individuals, many who wish to resist and liberate themselves from such conditions ultimately discover that it feels more like imprisonment followed by re-imprisonment. Despite being politically active, these subjects face severe political and social repercussions that often force them to retreat and cease their efforts.

The final characteristic of Real-Trauma is universalism. This concept extends beyond a moral framework applicable to everyone, as discussed by Kant in his liberal traditions. These traditional viewpoints advocate for global collective action driven by moral reasoning, aiming for perpetual peace. However, it is essential to note that the classical Kantian perspective, which should not be confused with the Kantian-Marxist perspective, does not address the challenges posed by anti-global capitalism. Additionally, universalism should not be equated with illegal actions often associated with imperial dominance and classical realism. Classical realism, in particular, is linked to Hobbesian ideas about international conflict, emphasizing the continuous struggle for power and the maintenance of dominance in global politics. Since the Kantian liberal paradigm may not adequately address the challenges presented by Hobbesian power dynamics today, a new form of universalism is being proposed. This new concept is referred to as Real-Trauma.

Real-Trauma is a concept that challenges the notions of universalism presented by Kant and Hobbes. It refers to a type of trauma that arises from recognizing global capitalism as a repressive force affecting everyone, regardless of differences in sexuality, race, or nationality. While Real-Trauma is an abstract idea, it manifests concretely as capitalist trauma. This form of trauma aligns with Marxist universalism and is connected to the Lacanian concept of the Real. Unlike Kant's and Hobbes's misleading universalisms, capitalist trauma reveals a stark, unpleasant reality that binds all subjects together without creating divisions. It also steers clear of the postcolonial focus on identity politics, which can lead many individuals to become overly fixated on localism, neglecting the broader implications of Real-Trauma.

Capitalist trauma is a dominant mode of existence that impacts individuals across diverse nations, races, genders, and languages, both in the Global North and in the Global South. This concept derives from the idea of Real-Trauma, which contrasts with Imaginary-Trauma, allowing the depoliticized proletariat individuals to see themselves as distinct from others, and Symbolic-Trauma, which supports identity politics and postcolonial perspectives. In essence, capitalist trauma is a tangible manifestation of the more abstract notion of Real-Trauma. Capitalist trauma is currently evident in various material forms, particularly through ongoing ecological and neo-colonial economic exploitation, overwhelming debt burdens, genocidal conflicts, and international wars, all of which are significant factors contributing to mass migration. Meanwhile, welfare programs are being drastically cut or nearly eliminated. This anti-capitalist trauma has become a top political priority. It is a universal issue that demands more urgent attention than the identity politics often emphasized by postcolonialism.

Capitalist trauma shares the characteristic of the Real-Trauma; it fills a void in the current understanding of trauma literature. Notably, there is a lack of a psychoanalytic critique of capitalism within the historiography of trauma studies, which has largely focused on cultural studies (Kaplan, 2005; Kaplan, 1990; Silverman, 1990; Neria and Ataria, 2016; Choi, 2020; Robson, 2022; Bounia and Witcomb, 2024), literary studies (Caruth, 2013; Caruth, 2016; Davis and Meretoja, 2020; Balaev, 2014; Kurtz, 2018; Trinidad, Çakırtaş, and Kızıltaş, 2018; Ganteau and Onega, 2013 and 2014; Ballengee and Kelman, 2021; Nadal and Calvo, 2014; Zilcosky, 2021), and history (Felman and Laub, 1992; Felman, 2002; Wieviorka, 2006; Bernard-Donals and Glejzer, 2003; LaCapra, 2001; Friedländer, 2007). Therefore, capitalist trauma aims to incorporate Lacanian psychoanalysis – a Lacanian theory of trauma – as a theory for a critique of capitalism. Many people living in the Global South continue to endure the repercussions of colonization and exploitation by the powerful nations. Žižek, who identifies as a moderately conservative communist and departs from postcolonial politics, observes that:

> Marx's metaphor for capital is the vampire, the parasitic, predatory living dead sucking the blood of the living – in the topsy-turvy world of capital, the dead rule over the living and are, in some ways, more alive than the living. The implicit premise (or promise) of this metaphor is that revolution would reverse this hierarchy – to upend the state of things and by doing so, return to the normal, 'natural' order in which the living rule over the dead.
>
> (Žižek, 2025b, p. 91)

For the proletariat, recognizing the trauma caused by capitalism is crucial. This acknowledgment is crucial for the political awareness of the proletariat, positioning them as a subject of resistance while also helping them understand their limitations. These limitations arise when the proletariat is overwhelmed by their own dialectical psyche. This presents a problem: while recognizing Real-Trauma may inspire the proletariat to become agents of resistance, the influence of Imaginary-Trauma and Symbolic-Trauma can dampen this desire, leading to a diminished motivation to challenge capitalism. In other words, this serves as a warning that the dialectical psyche of the proletariat creates challenges to Marx's focus on class consciousness, ultimately hindering the development of a unified class consciousness. Nonetheless, this issue can be deepened when the concept of capitalist trauma is integrated with dialectical materialism, focusing on both the connections and discrepancies between the two ideas. This topic will be explored further in the following section.

Existence: capitalist trauma in a critical dialogue with dialectical materialism

Dialectical materialism

For the proletariat, dialectical materialism is a fundamental philosophy of Marxism that emerged as a result of Marx's struggles against the right-wing followers of Hegel. This philosophy begins with a human reflection and an accurate understanding of the world, emphasizing that a social being exists as such. It distinguishes itself from idealism, which posits that the mind and the absolute ideal of the human spirit can be attained and are metaphysically situated outside the realities governing relationships among Men. In stark contrast to the right-wing interpretation that upholds the idealist aspects of Hegelian philosophy, Marx represents a left-wing Hegelianism by developing dialectical materialism. This philosophical approach starts from materialism itself, necessitating a critical examination of materialism to transform the conventional understanding of it and uncover the kernel of truth. Apropos of this, materialism reflects existing reality and aims to address human social production, highlighting the active role humans engage in creating things and the socio-economic relationships that arise from these activities. In essence, materialism signifies a tangible presence of social being, encompassing many individuals who identify with this socio-economic determinism.

According to Marx's philosophy, idealism fails to address a proper consciousness among people. He famously states, "It is not the consciousness of men that specifies their being, but on the contrary, their social being that specifies their consciousness" (Marx, 2021a, p. 160). This assertion, articulated by Marx, underscores not the philosophy of idealism but rather a finite correlation between existing objectivity – a social being – and the formation of human subjectivity. Marx's philosophy cannot be adequately understood by merely viewing subjectivity as a consciousness of social being. Instead, it is important to recognize that subjectivity takes on a concrete form, reflecting Marx's epistemological break from idealism. Materialism, as the foundation of human existence, does not operate on a naive notion of harmony. Rather, it is grounded in the internal contradictions that are inherent to social being. It is not possible to isolate a universal aspect of contradiction that fundamentally constitutes materialism. As Marx (2021a) asserts, "One must instead explain this consciousness from the contradictions of material life, from the already existing conflict between the forces of production and relations of production in society" (p. 160). This Marx's statement serves as the core principle of dialectics.

Dialectic is fundamentally a form of dialogue aimed at identifying opposing and conflictual aspects inherent to a specific matter. In materialism, which is inherently dialectical, internal contradictions naturally arise. This is a key aspect of dialectical materialism that aligns with Engels's thesis outlined in *Dialectics of Nature*. He first and foremost emphasizes the unity and struggle of opposites to illustrate a lack of unity in materialism and all material entities (Engels, 2025, p. 18). This indicates that all movements, actions, and motions in philosophical thought – including diverse branches of philosophy, science, mathematics, geometry – embody dynamics, reactions, and resistance, allowing this existing objectivism, as a replication of modernism, to shape and reshape an individual's subjectivity. Furthermore, Engels's concept of "the transformation of quantity into quality" signifies a gradual social change that culminates in significant socio-economic stages, such as feudalism, which gives rise to systemic injustices" (Engels, 2025, p. 18). This situation creates conditions ripe for a capitalist revolution, as exemplified by the French Revolution, driven by the bourgeoisie middle class. This process illustrates capitalism's ability to self-transform and perpetuate itself throughout history. Engels also introduces the idea of "the negation of negation", which highlights the limitations of existing realities (Engels, 2025, p. 20). The historical trajectory reveals that each new reality emerges from the previous one, but the new phase retains remnants of its predecessor. Thus, history, rather than being linear, is better represented as a spiral. In brief, according to Marx and Engels, dialectical materialism is a philosophy that reveals all phenomena as composed of opposing forces. The material world does not operate without flaws; historically, contradictions have been inherent in every aspect of materialism.

Capitalist trauma and dialectical materialism: a coordination between Lacanian and Marxist perspectives

Capitalist trauma can be theoretically linked to dialectical materialism. If capitalist trauma and dialectical materialism are understood as the current condition, it is crucial for the proletariat, as a subject of resistance, to separate itself from this condition (Lacan's *ex-sistence*). Otherwise, this existing situation will overwhelm and consume them. The task of philosophy is not merely to change the world blindly but to interpret it in a way that facilitates separation from it, ultimately enabling meaningful transformation. The connection between Marx and Lacan begins not directly with dialectical materialism but with materialism, which can be considered the "barred Other": a relationship between subjectivity and objectivity in the semblance of truth. Following this framework, materialism, or the human production of reality, serves as a semblance of truth. However, materialism, which involves the continuous production of goods, commodities, and products, reflects not just an animated reality but also conceals the Real-Trauma of capitalist exploitation. This exploitation manifests in two forms: direct exploitation (e.g., a proletariat being oppressed in the workplace) and indirect exploitation (such as a proletariat needing to provide financial support to unemployed family members), among other consequences.

Considering the concept of Real-Trauma, dialectical materialism implies that Marx does not merely invent a symptom reflecting the reality of materialism, specifically capitalism, but rather he parallels a psychoanalyst capable of identifying the Real-Trauma inherent in capitalism itself. Engels's proposal suggests a Lacanian notion of positive disavowal, distancing oneself from the semblance and fabrication of the true. This is because Engels's writings, to some extent, embody a radical logic of negation that opposes the illusory logic of capitalist perversion. Furthermore, materialism, which is concerned with the empty set (Ø), addresses the void at the center of its existence. To truly understand how materialism operates, it is essential to reconcile with the principle of dialectics and the act of negation put forth by Marx and Engels, while also recognizing the Real-Trauma within a Lacanian framework.

A communist fantasy: A discrepancy between Lacanian and Marxist perspectives

The conflicts between Lacanian and Marxist ideas become particularly clear when examining the concept of trauma. Marx focuses on dialectical materialism, emphasizing class consciousness and the transformation of current material conditions. However, as a non-psychoanalyst, he overlooks the trauma dimension that inherently involves dialectical reflection of the proletariat's complex existence. The existence of the proletariat within capitalism is not unitary; they experience overlapping and contradictory existential conditions.

To begin with, it is essential to discuss capitalist trauma, which arises from the realm of Real-Trauma and is distinct from Imaginary-Trauma. Imaginary-Trauma is inherently depoliticized and primarily centers on the individual's sense of self within the proletariat. For instance, a proletariat suffering from PTSD often feels alienated from their workplace and colleagues. In these cases, their main focus is on recovering from their mental health condition, seeking rehabilitation, and smoothly reintegrating into their work environment. As a result, they may recognize capitalism as a root cause of problems but may not perceive the need for class consciousness or a struggle against capitalism. Therefore, it is unreasonable for Marxists to expect or pressure a proletariat with PTSD to immediately develop class consciousness and rise against capitalism. Their ability to build solidarity and trust with fellow proletariats – both colleagues and strangers – is drastically diminished. Although those affected by PTSD may recognize the reality of capitalist trauma and the necessity to politically dismantle it, their actions do not necessarily aim to challenge the capitalist system directly. Rather than abolishing capitalism or seeking alternatives, they may engage in protests to address racial and sexual discrimination in workplaces and strive to document the history of these reforms for future generations. This emphasis on identity politics creates divisions among the proletariat based on race and sexuality, detracting from the possibility of a genuine Marxist revolution. Hence, amid the presence of Real-Trauma, there is a significant shift from Imaginary-Trauma to Symbolic-Trauma, which probably ends there. In other words, with Imaginary-Trauma (such as PTSD) and Symbolic-Trauma (such as identity politics), the efforts of the proletariat to overthrow the constraints of presentism, materialism, and the universalism characterized as capitalist trauma – the Real-Trauma – are even more difficult. Consequently, the proletariat encounters overlapping experiences – Real, Symbolic, and Imaginary Trauma – which intermingle and obstruct their ability to maintain a consistent stance on the abstract issues like the abolition of capitalism.

Moreover, there is a symptom of communist fantasy that continues as long as individuals believe that communism operates independently of the laws of dialectics. Dialectical materialism is connected to what Marx and Engels describe as "scientific socialism". To define this term, it is helpful to quote Engels at some length.

> To accomplish this act of universal emancipation is the historical mission of the modern proletariat. To thoroughly comprehend the historical conditions and thus the very nature of this act, to impart to the now oppressed proletariat

> class a full knowledge of the conditions and of the meaning of the momentous act it is called upon to accomplish, this is the task of the theoretical expression of the proletariat movement, scientific socialism.
>
> (Engels, 2004, p. 452)

This quality of scientific socialism resonates with Marx's statement that "communism is totally opposed to the existing world order" (Marx, 1998, p. 496).

In the context of scientific socialism, Engels privileges the proletariat revolution and envisions a communist world as a "solution of the contradictions". He asserts that "the proletariat seizes the public power" (Engels, 2004, p. 451) by transforming the privately held means of production of the capitalists into means of production that are socially distributed among everyone.

Arguably, the communist world attained by the proletariat revolution, envisioned by Marx and Engels, may ultimately be another form of communist fantasy rather than a true, non-dialectical society. It is unjust to critique capitalism or neoliberalism solely as a mere fantasy, asserting that it promises happiness to all based on the flawed principle of utilitarianism. It is equally fair and more important to recommend the idea of a communist fantasy. Therefore, for the sake of Lacanian psychoanalytical-philosophy concerning the question of truth, it is necessary to recognize that while neoliberalism is a fantasy, so too is communism.

Every ideological signifier is, at its core, a product of fantasy and a lack of coherency. At this point, it can be argued that this notion of scientific socialism represents a fantasy of Marxism infused with significant optimism. The essence of the proletariat argued throughout this book represents not only the alignment of Lacan and Marx but also a dissonance between the two thinkers. In other words, it is insufficient to address the intellectual partnership of Lacan and Marx in inventing a symptom of capitalism; instead, Lacan emerges as a thinker who creates a symptom relevant to Marx and Marxism.

Hence, in a Lacanian reflection – inventing a symptom to Marxism – there are six underlying aspects to address and raise awareness of a symptom of communist fantasy.

In the first aspect of communist fantasy, scientific socialism is the *telos* that challenges and transcends Lacanian enjoyment, which is typically understood in relation to an endless quest to fulfill a lack of desire within the oppressive framework of capitalism. Scientific socialism aims to move beyond the law of Lacanian enjoyment in order to reach a world that principally embodies universal freedom and the means of production accessible to all. However, this vision seems to be a communist fantasy. For the sake of egalitarianism and genuine emancipatory politics, Marx and Engels are likely to portray a scientifically utopian world free from the relentless human drive to satisfy endless desires – a drive often framed as Lacanian enjoyment within the matrical frontier of capitalism. This transformation can only occur when the proletariat "frees the means of production from the character of capital they have thus far borne, and gives their socialized character complete freedom to work itself out" (Engels, 2004, p. 451). Additionally, as previously quoted, the communist principle of "from each according to his abilities, to each according to his needs" exemplifies not only an ideal of complete freedom but also the universality of fulfilling desires. This principle, however, can violate the psychoanalytic notion of enjoyment for both capitalist and proletariat subjects. In Marx's conception of communism, Lacanian enjoyment is subverted, potentially leading to a world devoid of lack. This raises a debate regarding whether this idea of communism aligns with the nature of enjoyment described in psychoanalysis.

In the second aspect, Lacanian reflection urges the possibility that communism as a signifier cannot escape the Real. It may encounter the Real – the unsymbolized aspect of symptomatic elements that disrupt the entire fabric of reality. This suggests that the communist world may face disturbances, as what lies ahead could encompass the Real. The resolution of all contradictions should be viewed with skepticism; a belief in the communist world implies the existence of further unsymbolized contradictions. When the world of communism becomes the object of desire for the proletariat, the question arises: how can the proletariat ensure that this desired object that transcends the current capitalist Other – referred to as *objet a* – does not elude them? If a communist world is merely a signifier of the object of desire, it will inevitably confront the Real until it recognizes its own ontological incompletion. From a Lacanian perspective on signifiers, each signifier represents itself as another signifier. This idea reflects a Lacanian interpretation of a symptom within Marx's framework. Considering the Real-Trauma mentioned earlier, it is crucial to understand that the Real represents an absence; the unsurpassable. This implies that the Real will inevitably intervene in reality. A newly constructed reality, envisioned as a communist world, will ultimately confront this absence and its challenges, leading all of its members to experience alienation anew. The disruptive impact of the Real will not undermine the reality of a communist world from outside; rather, it will originate from within its own framework, causing damage and disintegration within such a utopian world eventually.

Third, the Marxist notion of dialectical materialism and scientific socialism emphasize an unreasonable and illegitimate distinction between the joy of the capitalist and the trauma of the proletariat. This binary opposition is fundamentally flawed and disregards the truth. It is significant to empirically acknowledge that some small- to medium-sized capitalists, such as those running SMEs and small groceries, also experience significant trauma and mental health issues; tragically, some have even taken their own lives during the COVID era. However, this suffering of capitalists is overlooked by Marxist scholars – intellectual elites in academia – who tend to focus exclusively on the plight of the proletariat. This leads to a distortion of truth. It is worth noting that capitalism dehumanizes and traumatizes not only the proletariat but also the capitalists. As noted in the introductory chapter, Lacan suggests that we are all proletariats, indicating that even capitalists are also proletarianized – dehumanized and traumatized – by the capitalist system.

In the fourth aspect, Marxist universalism tends to define the proletariat narrowly as those in relation to the social relation of economic production, as those who possess no means of production, viewing them as a group that is alienated and feels a lack of belonging within the capitalist system. This perspective represents another form of a communist fantasy. Such thinking is misleading because it implies that all capitalists feel a sense of belonging to capitalism. However, many capitalists also experience feelings of alienation from the system. Many seek psychological counseling, take leaves of absence, and feel traumatically pressured by the competitive environment and the time constraints of capitalism. This indicates that there are capitalists who also feel they do not ontologically belong within capitalism – a form of "lethal alienation" as mentioned in Chapter 3 – not just the proletariat.

In the fifth aspect, what Marxism fails to interrogate – an aspect often overlooked – is the relationship between capitalist subjects and their capital, such as businesses (factories, companies). The question is how capitalist subjects view their own capital? It is naive to believe that capitalists view their factories and companies only or primarily as sources of power, wealth, and profit. Relying on this symbolic interpretation – Symbolic appearance – alone creates a misleading impression – a false Imaginary – about the capitalists and their relationship with capital. As for the Real, many capitalists perceive and relate to their capital as a "prison". As long as their factories and companies can restrict their freedoms, resembling a "jail" from which they cannot escape – a trauma – as doing so would leave them with nothing to live for.

In the sixth aspect, it is presupposed that a communist society establishes a trustworthy superstructure that others will follow. In other words, a communist society seeks to build trust within its new superstructure before encouraging collective trust among the proletariat, the human members of society. However, emphasizing trust in this way is an entire pitfall. The problem is that trust should not be considered a crucial foundational element of a communist society.

Trust should not be promoted as a political factor for communism or for the formation of a superstructure where everyone follows the same path; this is a communist fantasy. Liberal institutionalism and international frameworks also rely on the concept of trust as a superstructure. When this liberal system is challenged by the power of exceptional imperialism and by oligarchs advocating for a post-liberal order (Deneen, 2024) – one that seeks to undermine trust in liberalism, its legal framework, and global norms, domestically, while promoting global conflicts to accelerate geopolitical competitions – trust fostered in the liberal order as a superstructure collapses. Promoting trust as a political factor is self-detrimental. Additionally, Marx's authentic vision of communism – not the quasi-Marxism represented by bourgeois-style democratic socialism, which is often promoted by leftist elites and academia – envisions a society characterized by four essential elements:

(a) A classless society, in which there is no hierarchical order, and a sufficiency of want and a necessity is shared and enjoyed equally by all. This is what Marx thematizes, "actual enjoyment of existence" that represents "universal consciousness" that is equated with "a totality of human manifestations of life" (Marx, 2007, p. 81);
(b) A propertyless society, where private ownership is abolished, and everyone collectively owns the means of production to produce and circulate vital items and things based on their abilities and needs (Marx, 2007, p. 79);
(c) A stateless society, where the state temporarily ruled by the "dictatorship of the proletariat" (Marx, 2021b, p. 222) that represents true republic, eventually withers away, allowing society to govern itself based on the principle of autonomy as part of subjectivity prompt with a new mode of objectivity such as "local municipal liberty" (Marx, 2021c, p. 186) – Marx is typically a non-statist political theorist and this means that Vladimir Lenin and Mao-Tsetung are the representative of quasi-Marxist pragmatists insofar as they are state-centric pragmatists;
(d) A moneyless society, in which all individuals become "a working man, and productive labor ceases to be a class attribute" (Marx, 2021c, p. 187). This is a "working-class government" in which everyone – capitalists, the rich, and the poor in the old capitalist world – ideally transforms into working man, where all members in the new communist world can share, care, and generously exchange goods as use-value without money as exchange-value, contributing to the entire flourish of the communist society.

The four foundational characteristics of a communist society present an alternative to the current capitalist world. However, this vision seems unconvincing and cannot be realized without fostering trust among the proletariat and prioritizing the overall spiritual growth of the subject. Many scholars and activists often advocate for democratic socialism as a substitute for Marx's genuine vision of communism. Arguably, in the present, it is difficult to find a true, traditional Marxist theorist who adheres to Marx's original theses as a German Kantian communist dialectical materialist philosopher. Moreover, the key to achieving a communist society may lie in cultivating what psychoanalysis refers to as free association among the hysterical proletariat, despite their internal struggles. However, this potential internal disruption caused by free association among the proletariat could impede the development of a communist society. Therefore, it is unrealistic to envision a communist society as a solution to all contradictions without carefully considering all six aspects already mentioned.

Embracing dangers: the proletariat as a post-traumatic subject

Marx defines the proletariat primarily through the lens of labor and surplus-value, viewing them as individuals who exchange their labor for wages. In a non-psychoanalytical perspective, the term "proletariat" is determined by social relationships, particularly in the economic context, where it refers to those who lack ownership of the means of production. Furthermore, Marx believes that proletariat is a chief political agent for liberation and emancipation. This understanding is replicated and consistent with traditional Marxist thought.

However, this understanding of the proletariat does not address a psychoanalytical question: what is the essence of the subjectivity of the proletariat within a communist framework? The question that Marx abandons is thus: how can one psychoanalytically define the life form of the proletariat in the vision of communism? In other words, Marx fails to elaborate on what the life experience of a proletariat subject would be in relation to a communist society.

Exploring this concept through Lacanian trauma theory enhances the understanding of Marx's view on the communist world, which centers on the relationship between the proletariat and their subjectivity. In a communist context, it is possible that a new type of subject emerges as the post-traumatic subject. This subject actively chooses freedom while also confronting the inherent risks of facing dangers but enjoys embracing it. Unlike individuals suffering from PTSD, this subject can be seen as a non-meaningful signifier within the ideological landscape shaped by capitalist trauma.

The post-traumatic subject refers to proletariats who are not weakened by mental illness. Specifically, this subject embodies the proletariat in an unstable mental state, armed with a global resistance ideology against capitalist trauma. With this political aim in mind, the post-traumatic subject is, to some extent, one that lacks symbolic status; however, this does not imply that the subject is forced to abandon the symbolic order. Rather, it is a subject that actively chooses to sever ties with the existing order due to its oppressive nature, which perpetuates the recurrence of Real-Trauma. This political subject embraces danger, rejecting the subjugation of capitalist ideologies that permeate universal trauma: this form of proletariat subjectivity is different from signifying them as individuals whose life is processed and commoditized into a surplus-value.

Additionally, the proletariat as a post-traumatic subject understands that true recovery from mental illness cannot depend solely on clinical settings and therapeutic techniques. For genuine political emancipation – beyond simply recovering from a dire health condition dominated by the psychoanalyst's medical knowledge – a universal global force must be mobilized on behalf of the proletariat to combat capitalist trauma, enabling a recovery from mental illness at the same time. This post-traumatic subject is akin to the hysterical subject, which is poised to pave the way for a communist future. However, before achieving full freedom in this new world, this subject has to embrace dangers. The essential characteristic of a post-traumatic subject can be illustrated by referencing Lacan's observations:

> *Your money or your life!* If I choose the money, I lose both. If I choose life, I have life without the money, namely a life deprived of something. I think I have made myself clear.
>
> (Lacan, 1981b, p. 212; italics original)

Following Lacan, when a proletariat "chooses money", such as wages and salaries offered by a capitalist – whether an employer or a current boss – this choice is not dangerous but can lead to unpleasant outcomes. There are two main consequences to consider for this safe option. First, the proletariat may experience a loss of money due to exploitation by other capitalists, such as debt repayment or rent for housing. Additionally, the proletariat must struggle with the current inflation rate and the high prices set by other capitalists in the market, which can quickly deplete their finances and deprive them of enjoyment. Second, the proletariat's life may be diminished because the capitalist system presents itself as the desire of the Other. This leads the proletariat to realize, often uncomfortably, that their existence revolves around conforming to the desires of capitalism. These outcomes define characteristics of capitalist trauma that affect the proletariat.

If the proletariat, as a post-traumatic subject, begins to choose a life of their own, they will gain freedom and experience "life without money", as this is the essence of embracing dangers. For example, if they choose to resist capitalism politically through actions like work strikes and protests, they intend to deprive it of their symbolic status within the capitalist framework. However, this conscious decision to forgo their symbolic status is not only a preliminary step in challenging capitalism but also a fundamental aspect of freedom connected to their courage in embracing death, as Lacan suggests, "You choose freedom. Well! You've got freedom to die" (Lacan, 1981b, p. 213). Marx and Engels, not being psychoanalysts, do not fully recognize the proletariat as an embodiment of the post-traumatic subject. From a psychoanalytic viewpoint, a post-traumatic subject, when significantly represented in the life of the proletariat, reflects an ethical struggle for freedom while also grappling with an encouragement in embracing dangers and other unpleasant consequences, including the challenges posed by capitalism that they are likely to face.

A Lacanian understanding of subjectivity does not view the subject as a single, unified entity. Instead, it posits that the proletariat, who seeks liberation from the Real-Trauma associated with capitalism, can be analyzed psychoanalytically as a post-traumatic subject – an aspect that Marx and Engels did not envision. However, this category of proletariat can be disrupted by Symbolic-Trauma, which may hinder their quest for liberation from capitalist trauma. This disruption can lead them to see postcolonial politics and radical democracy – Laclauian politics – as alternatives, diverting them from the revolutionary path. Additionally, they may also be affected by their own mental health issues, termed Imaginary-Trauma, which can further limit their development as post-traumatic subjects: the subject that dares to embrace pain, isolation, alienation, and ultimately dangers. Consequently, it is challenging for the proletariat to achieve a cohesive post-traumatic subjectivity; their experience is often characterized by a fragmented nature, complicating the formation of their subjectivities.

Proletariat and the politics of trauma: beyond postcolonialism and identity politics

Capitalist trauma represents the material condition in which all subjects exist: this is a universal presenting material condition that affects everyone. This critical reflection is rational because capitalist trauma has manifested through various economic crises, such as the Asian Financial Crisis of 1997 and the Global Financial Crisis of 2008, which have impacted everyone. At this stage, postcolonial politics should extend beyond merely addressing local trauma and identity formation related to collective memory, particularly for indigenous populations in the Global South who have experienced displacement at borders. It should also actively engage in the crucial task of challenging the trauma of capitalist system, which is perpetuated by geopolitical competition and domination. To effectively address these issues on a global scale, it is possible for one to seek a genuine form of emancipatory politics that intertwines anti-colonialism with anti-capitalism. However, the significant challenge for the proletariat is forming a unified post-traumatic subjectivity as a means of resisting capitalist trauma, although this may not always be achievable.

Before the emergence of capitalist trauma, there was a trauma of postcolonialism, which represents a collective experience stemming from the shared suffering of formerly colonized nations. However, capitalist trauma goes beyond the traumas associated with postcolonialism, provincialism, and localism. Unlike the trauma of postcolonialism, which is often tied to specific non-Western cultural contexts, capitalist trauma aims to unify individual proletariats from both the Global North and Global South. It emphasizes trauma featuring as universality (Supachalasai, 2014). In essence, capitalist trauma seeks to map and articulate the pain and suffering of a universal proletariat rather than focusing solely on the distressing memories of indigenous peoples in particular regions, such as borderlands and riverine areas. The intellectual challenge posed by a hypothesis, trauma as a political factor, lies in its opposition to the emphasis on enjoyment that is inherent in capitalism – an emphasis that shapes social relationships and often accentuates desire and lack tied to the surplus-enjoyment of the capitalist framework. The discussion here shifts away from the impossible fulfillment of profit rates and commodity production, realized as enjoying the lack, in the capitalist system.

This psychoanalytic critique of capitalism, inspired by Lacan's concept of enjoyment, successfully shifts the focus from the traditional Marxist emphasis on surplus-value. However, it does not free everyone from the constraints of capitalism. The capitalist system is often marked by a lack of genuine desire and an excess of enjoyment, which frequently reflects the insatiable greed of the bourgeoisie and their luxurious, self-indulgent lifestyles rooted in dissatisfaction with the present. When discussing the benefits of capitalism and the enjoyment it provides, it is crucial to consider other economic factors, such as inflation and household debt faced by the proletariat in both developed and developing countries. These factors often lead to a halt in the proletariat's enjoyment. This suggests that relying on enjoyment as a political factor – when introduced as a new element for critiquing capitalism – tends to merely reflect how capitalism operates. Unfortunately, this discussion overlooks other psychoanalytical experiences of the proletariat in the analysis unless enjoyment is connected to the specific experiences of the proletariat, as addressed in Chapter 4 of this book.

Nonetheless, the concept of universal trauma is closely linked to capitalistic experiences, suggesting that the proletariat must shed their current material conditions. This suggests that the proletariat can be seen as a post-traumatic subject, despite potential inconsistencies in this formation of subjectivity. However, postcolonial literature often focuses on historical events such as civil wars, crackdowns, and genocides within the context of colonialism, neglecting to address the aspect of capitalist trauma. Many distressing memories from countries in the previously colonized Global South challenge the Global North's emphasis on imperial memory, such as the remembrance of the Holocaust and September 11. These postcolonial memories reflect a multiplicity of suffering, feelings of unbelonging, self-reflections, remembrance, and narratives that are rooted in indigenous perspectives. These narratives center on postcolonial tenets and diverge from Western viewpoints. Trauma studies, influenced by a rhetoric of difference in postcolonial contexts, tend to be highly divisive and contextually specific (Craps, 2013; Rajiva, 2021; Zapata, 2021; Romdhani and Tunca, 2022; Ward, 2015; Karmakar and Khan, 2023; Gairola and Jayawickrama, 2021). Notable examples of this relationship can be found in scholarly works concerning the Vietnam War (Pelley, 2002), Cambodia (Loughlin, 2024), and the October 6 massacre and protests against the government in Thailand (Winichakul, 2020). As long as capitalist trauma seeks to create a universal understanding of the suffering experienced by the proletariat in both the Global North and Global South, this concept differs significantly from the binary oppositions represented by imperialism of memory and resistance in postcolonial trauma and cultural constructions and reconstructions. For the sake of emancipatory politics, it is worth referencing the words of Žižek as follows:

> In today's triumph of global capitalism, the argument goes, true resistance is not possible, so all we can do till the revolutionary spirit of the global working class is renewed is defend what remains of the welfare state, confronting those in power with demands we know they cannot fulfil, and otherwise withdraw into cultural studies, where one can quietly pursue the work of criticism.

> Or, it takes the 'postmodern' route, shifting the accent from anti-capitalist struggle to the multiple forms of politico-ideological struggle for hegemony, emphasizing the importance of discursive re-articulation.
>
> (Žižek, 2007)

Soravis Jayanama entails this debate; his warning is that so many people these days are familiar with "apocalyptic fetishism"; they know the catastrophe is coming and unavoidable, but they act as if nothing happens (pp. 373–419). Jayanama's caution corresponds with Jean-Pierre Dupuy's statement, precisely, "if there are economic chaos and social unrest, this will be necessary and inevitable, we could change the frame itself within which our fate seems predetermined" (Dupuy as cited in Žižek, 2025a, p. 105). Žižek then engenders this point eventually with the question: "but what if we remain faithful to the Leftist tradition and maintain the solidarity of those who rebel?" (Žižek, 2023a, p. 77). In Žižek's politics opposable to identity politics, the solidarity of the Leftist tradition is different from Ernesto Laclau's Left populism. "The Left populism should construct a different figure of the Enemy, not the threatening racial Other (immigrant, Jew, Muslim . . .) but the financial elites, fundamentalists, and other 'usual suspects' of the progressives" (Žižek, 2020, p. 285). This solidarity against financial oligarchy is a political legacy that is worth fighting for. He also continues that "today, the ultimate "enemy" is not a concrete social agent but in some sense the [capitalist/financial] system itself, a certain functioning of the system, which cannot be easily located into agents" (Žižek, 2020, p. 285).

In *Too Late to Awaken* (2023), Žižek (2023b) suggests that "let's mobilize ourselves to attack the roots of our crisis, with all the risks that this involves. Because the greatest risk today is doing nothing and allowing history to follow its course" (p. 164). Following Žižek, one should not be overly optimistic about the subject of resistance and traditional Left solidarity, because the politics of the proletariat aimed at challenging capitalist trauma appear to encounter ontological inconsistencies regarding their divided subjectivity. In other words, it is important to acknowledge that the proletariat – as a post-traumatic subject that Marx, Engels, and traditional Marxism did not foresee this aspect of trauma inherent to the proletariat – requires to analyze and reveal the root cause of the crisis: capitalist trauma. Assumed as a post-traumatic subject, they have to take significant risks to reach a world where they can feel a stronger sense of belonging and experience less alienation, in contrast to the capitalist trauma that has left them dispossessed and extremely alienated. The question remains: do they have the courage not to derail from such progress and to form an ontological consistency regarding solidarity, in which their subjectivities must struggle against the internal dynamics of dialecticism?

In conclusion, Lacan's concepts of the RSI inform a nuanced theory of trauma, proposing that trauma is a significant political factor. This framework distinguishes three types of traumas: Imaginary-Trauma, Symbolic-Trauma, and

Real-Trauma, which are related to capitalist trauma. Imaginary-Trauma leads the proletariat to form subjectivities based on self-perception, which may contribute to depoliticization through reliance on medical care. In contrast, Real-Trauma, or capitalist trauma, differs from Symbolic-Trauma, where the proletariat articulates symbolic identity politics, focusing on the abolition of gender and racial prejudices, but risks neglecting a critique of capitalism. Despite theoretical differences with Marx's dialectical materialism, the three trauma types are interconnected, highlighting complexity in proletariat subjectivity. It is crucial to view the proletariat not just as labor entities but as post-traumatic subjects willing to confront existing social structures and courageous to embrace dangers.

The ideas of capitalist trauma and the proletariat as a post-traumatic subject can foster important discussions opposable to postcolonial and Laclauian politics. This view emphasizes that a universal approach to emancipatory politics needs a critique of capitalism. Ultimately, challenges arise and inevitably remain when efforts to challenge capitalism rely on the proletariat, given the complexities of proletariat subjectivity. Proletariats experiencing capitalist trauma understand the need to oppose capitalism but may struggle to initiate revolution. Instead, they might regress into Imaginary-Trauma (a feeling that proletariat solidarity is unattainable) and Symbolic-Trauma (viewing proletariat politics as identity politics), complicating their path to revolutionary action. This creates a challenging mental struggle for them, enduring a dialectical psychical condition.

Reference list

Balaev, M. (2014). *Contemporary Approaches in Literary Trauma Theory*. London Borough of Camden: Palgrave Macmillan.

Ballengee, J., and David Kelman. (2021). *Trauma and Literature in an Age of Globalization*. Oxon and New York: Routledge.

Bernard-Donals, M., and Richard Glejzer. (2003). *Essays on Representation and the Holocaust*. London and Wisconsin: The University of Wisconsin Press.

Bounia, A., and Andrea Witcomb. (2024). *The Ethics of Collecting Trauma: The Role of Museums in Collecting and Displaying Contemporary Crises*. Oxon and New York: Routledge.

Caruth, C. (2013). *Literature in the Ashes of History*. Maryland: Johns Hopkins University Press.

Caruth, C. (2016). *Unclaimed Experience: Trauma, Narrative, and History*. Twentieth Anniversary Edition. Baltimore: Johns Hopkins University Press.

Choi, C. (2020). *Healing Historical Trauma in South Korean Film and Literature*. London and New York: Routledge.

Craps, S. (2013). *Postcolonial Witnessing: Trauma Out of Bounds*. Hampshire and New York: Palgrave Macmillan.

Davis, C., and Hanna Meretoja. (2020). *The Routledge Companion to Literature and Trauma*. London and New York: Routledge.

Deneen, P. (2024). *Regime Change: Towards a Postliberal Future*. New York: Forum.

Derrida, J. (1994). *Specters of Marx: The State of the Debt, the Work of Mourning, and the New International*. London and New York: Routledge.

Engels, F. (2004). 'Socialism: Utopian and Scientific', in *Karl Marx: Essential Thinkers*. London: CRW Publishing Limited.
Engels, F. (2025). 'Dialectics', in *Dialectics of Nature*. Zinc Read.
Felman, S. (2002). *The Juridical Unconscious: Trials and Traumas in the Twentieth Century*. Cambridge, Massachusetts, and London: Harvard University Press.
Felman, S., and Dori Laub. (1992). *Testimony: Crises of Witnessing in Literature, Psychoanalysis, and History*. Oxon and New York: Routledge.
Friedländer, S. (2007). *The Years of Extermination: Nazi Germany and the Jews, 1939–1945*. New York: HarperCollins.
Gairola, R., and Sharanya Jayawickrama. (2021). *Memory, Trauma, Asia: Recall, Affect, and Orientalism in Contemporary Narratives*. Oxon and New York: Routledge.
Ganteau J-M., and Susana Onega. (2013). *Trauma and Romance in Contemporary British Literature*. Oxon and New York: Routledge.
Ganteau J-M., and Susana Onega. (2014). *Contemporary Trauma Narratives: Liminality and the Ethics of Form*. Oxon and New York: Routledge.
Jayanama, S. (2022). *Everything You Always Wanted to Know about Global Politics but Were Afraid to Ask Lacan* [in Thai]. Bangkok: Siam Publishing House.
Kaplan, A. (1990). *Psychoanalysis & Cinema*. London and New York: Routledge.
Kaplan, A. (2005). *Trauma Culture: The Politics of Terror and Loss in Media and Literature*. New Brunswick, New Jersey, and London. Rutgers University Press.
Karmakar, G., and Zeenat Khan. (2023). *Narratives of Trauma in South Asian Literature*. New York and Oxon: Routledge.
Kurtz, R. (2018). *Trauma and Literature*. Cambridge: Cambridge University Press.
Lacan, J. (1974). *Le Séminaire XXII. R.S.I.* (1974–1975), texte établi par Jacques-Alain Miller, *Ornicar?,* 1975(2) (seminar of 10 December 1974).
Lacan, J. (1981a). 'From Interpretation to the Transference', in *The Seminar of Jacques Lacan Book XI: The Four Fundamental Concepts of Psychoanalysis*. Edited by Jacques Alain-Miller. Translated by Alan Sheridan. London and New York: W.W. & Norton Company.
Lacan, J. (1981b). 'The Subject and the Other: Alienation', in *The Seminar of Jacques Lacan Book XI: The Four Fundamental Concepts of Psychoanalysis*. Edited by Jacques Alain-Miller. Translated by Alan Sheridan. London and New York: W.W. & Norton Company.
Lacan, J. (1981c). 'The Subject and the Other: Aphanisis', in *The Seminar of Jacques Lacan Book XI: The Four Fundamental Concepts of Psychoanalysis*. Edited by Jacques Alain-Miller. Translated by Alan Sheridan. London and New York: W.W. & Norton Company
Lacan, J. (1991). 'Discourse Analysis and Ego Analysis', in *The Seminar of Jacques Lacan Book I: Freud's Papers on Technique*. Edited by Jacques-Alain Miller. Translated by John Forrester. London and New York: W.W. & Norton Company.
Lacan, J. (1999a). 'Knowledge and Truth', in *The Seminar of Jacques Lacan Book XX: Encore: On Feminine Sexuality, The Limits of Love and Knowledge*. Edited by Jacques-Alain Miller. Translated by Bruce Fink. London and New York: W.W. & Norton Company.
Lacan, J. (1999b). 'To Jakobson', in *The Seminar of Jacques Lacan Book XX: Encore: On Feminine Sexuality, The Limits of Love and Knowledge*. Edited by Jacques-Alain Miller. Translated by Bruce Fink. London and New York: W.W. & Norton Company.
Lacan, J. (2006a). 'Seminar on "The Purloined Letter"', in *Écrits: The First Complete Edition in English*. Translated by Bruce Fink. London and New York: W.W. & Norton Company.

Lacan, J. (2006b). 'The Subversion of the Subject and the Dialectic of Desire in the Freudian Unconscious', in *Écrits: The First Complete Edition in English*. Translated by Bruce Fink. London and New York: W.W. & Norton Company.
LaCapra, D. (2001). *Writing History, Writing Trauma*. Baltimore: Johns Hopkins University Press.
Laclau, E., and Chantal Mouffe. (2001). *Hegemony and Socialist Strategy: Towards a Radical Democratic Politics*. 2nd Edition. London and New York: Verso.
Loughlin, N. (2024). *The Politics of Coercion: State and Regime Making in Cambodia*. Cornell: Cornell University Press.
Marx, K. (1998). 'Critique of German Socialism According to Its Various Prophets', in *The German Ideology*. New York: Prometheus Books.
Marx, K. (2007). 'From the Paris Notebook', in *Marx Early Political Writings*. Edited and Translated by Joseph O'Malley. Cambridge: Cambridge University Press.
Marx, K. (2021a). 'A Contribution to the Critique of Political Economy', in *Marx Later Political Writings*. Edited and Translated by Terrell Carver. Cambridge and New York: Cambridge University Press.
Marx, K. (2021b). 'Critique of the Gotha Programme', in *Marx Later Political Writings*. Edited and Translated by Terrell Carver. Cambridge and New York: Cambridge University Press.
Marx, K. (2021c). 'The Civil War in France', in *Marx Later Political Writings*. Edited and Translated by Terrell Carver. Cambridge and New York: Cambridge University Press.
Nadal, M., and Mónica Calvo. (2014). *Trauma in Contemporary Literature: Narrative and Representation*. Oxon and New York: Routledge.
Neiman, S. (2023). *Left is not Woke*. Cambridge and Hoboken: Polity Press.
Neria, Y., and Yochai Ataria. (2016). 'Trauma and Culture: How Trauma and Shape the Human Mind', in *Interdisciplinary Handbook of Trauma and Culture*. Edited by Yochai Ataria, David Gurevitz, Haviva Pedaya, and Yuval Neria. Switzerland: Springer International Publishing.
Peck, W., Charles Drebing, and Russell Schutt. (2002). 'PTSD in the Workplace', in *Handbook of Mental Health in the Workplace*. Edited by Jay Thomas and Michel Hersen. London: Sage Publications.
Pelley, P. (2002). *Postcolonial Vietnam: New Histories of the National Past*. Durham and London: Duke University Press.
Rajiva, J. (2021). *Towards an Animist Reading of Postcolonial Trauma Literature*. Oxon and New York: Routledge.
Robson, K. (2022). *Writing Wounds: The Inscription of Trauma in Post-1968 French Women's Life-writing*. Leiden: Brill Publishers.
Romdhani, R., and Daria Tunca. (2022). *Narrating Violence in the Postcolonial World*. Oxon and New York: Routledge.
Silverman, K. (1990). 'Male Subjectivity at the Margins', in *Psychoanalysis & Cinema*. Edited by Ann Kaplan. London and New York: Routledge.
Supachalasai, C. (2014). 'A Trauma Revisited: Fanon, Žižek, and Violence', *International Journal of Žižek Studies*, 8(2)
Supachalasai, C. (2017). *Theorising the Politics of Survivor: Memory, Trauma, and Subjectivity in International Politics*. PhD Thesis Submitted to Department of International Politics. Aberystwyth University.
Trinidad, A., Önder Çakırtaş, and Şahin Kızıltaş. (2018). *The Politics of Traumatic Literature: Narrating Human Psyche and Memory*. E-book. Cambridge Scholars Publishing.
Ward, A. (2015). *Postcolonial Traumas: Memory, Narrative, Resistance*. New York and Hampshire: Palgrave Macmillan.

Wieviorka, A. (2006). *The Era of the Witness*. Translated by Jared Stark. Ithaca and London: Cornell University Press.
Winichakul, T. (2020). *Moments of Silence: The Unforgetting of the October 6, 1976, Massacre in Bangkok*. Honolulu: University of Hawai'i Press.
Zapata, B. (2021). *Zadie Smith and Postcolonial Trauma: Decolonising Trauma, Decolonising Selves*. London and New York: Routledge.
Zilcosky, J. (2021). *The Language of Trauma: War and Technology in Hoffman, Freud, and Kafka*. Toronto, Buffalo and London: University of Toronto Press.
Žižek, S. (2007). 'Resistance is Surrender', *London Review of Books*. 29(22). https://www.lrb.co.uk/the-paper/v29/n22/slavoj-zizek/resistance-is-surrender. Accessed: October 10, 2025.
Žižek, S. (2020). 'Which Idea of Europe is Worth Defending?', *Crisis and Critique: The Future of Europe*. 7(1), 278–293.
Žižek, S. (2023a). 'Against the Solidarity of Those in Power', in *Too Late to Awaken: What Lies Ahead When There is no Future*. London: Penguin Books.
Žižek, S. (2023b). 'Conclusion: How Do We Begin When It's Too Late?', in *Too Late to Awaken: What Lies Ahead When There Is No Future*. London: Penguin Books.
Žižek, S. (2025a). 'Disavowal', in *Against Progress*. London and New York: Bloomsbury Academic.
Žižek, S. (2025b). 'We Are Biomass', in *Against Progress*. London and New York: Bloomsbury Academic.

8 Proposing a Lacanian formula for proletariat discourse

What is proletariat discourse?

Proletariat discourse is a psychoanalytical-political exploration of the speculative truth of the proletariat from a Lacanian perspective. In this context, the term "discourse" does not relate to power and knowledge in the Foucauldian sense. Instead, it emphasizes the formation of statements and the speech acts that seek to map and speculate on the truth of the proletariat. This idea originated from the global protest movements on different issues, such as anti-austerity, anti-authoritarianism, and anti-war, joined by the proletariat that occurred between 2019 and 2025 in various countries. During these events, the engagement of the proletariat became readily apparent. These global events prompted a philosophical question: what is the proletariat? What is the truth of the proletariat? Upon reflection, it recognizes the difficulty of grasping the diverse historical formations of the proletariat across the globe. Given the limitations of history, time, and space, it becomes clear that formulating a universal narrative about the proletariat is impossible. Thus, the thesis of this book opts for a speculative approach to understanding the truth of the proletariat through a Lacanian psychoanalytic lens. Consequently, this discourse can also be referred to as a "Lacanian Proletariat". As long as Lacan's discourse laws do not simply represent a social bond, all elements of knowledge within the discourse are epistemologically open to debate, dialectical reflection, and constructive engagement. Proletariat discourse is not exempt from this rule established by Lacan.

Why proletariat discourse?

There are two key reasons why engaging in proletariat discourse is necessary. First, the concept of the proletariat seems to align with the perspectives of the late Lacan, referring to his psychoanalytic thoughts and developments after the May 1968 student and worker uprising in Paris, France. The term "proletariat" appears occasionally in Lacan's discussions and seminars, almost as if it were a slip of the tongue, revealing Lacan's unconscious desire. Although he referenced

DOI: 10.4324/9781003657781-8

Marx's idea of the proletariat in several seminars, he never had the opportunity to dedicate a session specifically to this topic. It seems that the concept of the proletariat occupied Lacan's thoughts during the time; however, he did not fully develop his understanding of proletariat discourse before his death in 1981. Hence, in the past, Lacan invented the capitalist discourse, but it is necessary to focus on developing and advancing the proletariat discourse in the present.

The late Lacan was interested in Marx's theories of surplus-value and, certainly, the proletariat, but approached it with caution. While Lacan's notion of "exit from capitalist discourse" has some similarities with Marx's idea of proletariat revolution, it is essential to approach the application of Lacan's psychoanalysis to Marxist revolutionary politics with careful consideration. Lacan should not be equated with communism or Marxism. Lacan's perspective can challenge any socially constructed signifiers, including those relating to Marxist politics. According to Lacanian psychoanalysis, every signifier – whether it pertains to Marxist revolutionary politics or the concept of a communist society – must address its own inherent flaws and contradictions. Lacan tends to be skeptical of both right-wing and left-wing ideologies. It is notable that during his lifetime, he never officially aligned himself with either faction; he is typically beyond the political spectrum of Left and Right.

Second, the proletariat discourse incorporates both Lacan's and Marx's theories, emphasizing their commonalities and differences in discussing the proletariat while avoiding a bias of sameness between the two thinkers. Through the lens of Lacanian psychoanalysis, the question posed by Marxism is thus: how can Lacanian psychoanalysis enhance Marxist critiques of capitalism and political revolution? The typical response revolves around the intention to utilize Lacanian psychoanalysis as a critical framework that supports and aligns with revolutionary ideals of traditional Marxism. In other words, this approach raises valid concerns about the potential for psychoanalysis to be interpreted in a way that is used to support Marxist notions. This Lacanian-Marxist trajectory begins by illustrating the proletariat revolution or the proletariat subject as the traumatic Real: a site of antagonism against capitalism. In this sense, capitalism represents a fantasy governed by the pleasure principle, driven not just by surplus-value but also by surplus-enjoyment. In contrast, political correctness and identity politics symbolize a form of Symbolic tribalism that diverts attention from the Real essence of the proletariat revolution and a critique of capitalism. As a result, the Imaginary suggests an illusion where it appears that nothing is changing, even as conditions progress toward a state of great downfall.

This perspective tends to reinforce traditional Marxist thinking, suggesting that Lacanian psychoanalysis and conventional Marxism – Lacan and Marx – are aligned in their revolutionary pursuits. Ultimately, this implies that Lacan is fundamentally Marxist, representing the old Left rather than the inverse. In this trajectory, Marx is not only a thinker who invents a symptom of capitalism, but Lacan and Marx also mutually invent a symptom of capitalism, despite their different conceptual frameworks. Despite this intellectual – silent partnership – between Marx and Lacan, some Marxists might argue that psychoanalysis is unhelpful to them because it often interprets Marx's ideas using its own Lacanian terminology. This approach tends to overlook any weaknesses in Marx's theories and does not offer new insights into Marxist thought.

Hence, the question arises regarding how Lacan introduces a critical perspective to traditional Marxism. How does Lacan create a symptom for Marx? Psychoanalysis should reposition itself not only to foster a partnership with Marxism but also to introduce skepticism, limitations, disparities, and new insights into Marx's theories. When rethinking Marx's concept of the proletariat, it is necessary to consider how Lacanian psychoanalysis can identify limitations and unconscious assumptions that Marx himself may not have recognized. In the proletariat discourse, the objective is to revisit Marx through the lens of Lacan as a critical theorist: it is not merely a matter of placing Lacan alongside Marx but also of positioning Lacan in constructive opposition to Marx in order to further develop Marxist theory. This approach could be beneficial, particularly in stimulating intellectual thinking and inspiration. For instance, while Marx is commonly signified or viewed by traditional Marxist as revolutionary thinker, this signifier may be insufficient and reveals a lack from a Lacanian psychoanalytic perspective. Why not try to redefine Marx using Lacan's four discourses? The outcome of this redefinition might be as follows:

1. Master Discourse: In this discourse, Marx appears as a leader in the revolutionary movement – a proponent of the function of class struggle – aiming to challenge bourgeois ideology and socialism.
2. University Discourse: Here, Marx is depicted as an author of books and pamphlets, advocating for his doctrines to his followers such as traditional Marxist scholars and university students. The academic interpretation of Marx – a standard for reading him correctly by distinguishing it from those who have misunderstood his work – strengthens elitist scholars, journal publications, and the bourgeois university.
3. Hysterical Discourse: In this context, Marx opposes capitalism and expresses his unconscious desires related to the communist utopia.
4. Analyst Discourse: Finally, this portrayal of Marx's interaction with the proletariat realizes how the proletariat is exploited and oppressed within a capitalist society, positioning Marx as an analyst and the proletariat as the analysand.

These four dimensions illustrate that Marx encompasses multiple perspectives. It is through this psychoanalytical understanding that traditional Marxism can expand its theoretical framework, recognizing the debt it owes to psychoanalysis. This complex line of thinking offers an example of how psychoanalysis can enrich Marxism, encouraging the development of Marxist theory. To reiterate, it is crucial to highlight an ontological rift between Lacan and Marx, emphasizing the depth of this discussion.

A Lacanian formula for proletariat discourse

Proletariat discourse exists as an unconscious element within capitalist discourse. It forms a kind of non-relationship – something that is always present within capitalist thought, yet remains unspoken and repressively unexamined. In simpler terms, proletariat discourse represents the *objet a* – the point of ontological excess that already exists within capitalist discourse. Proletariat discourse or a Lacanian understanding of the proletariat aims to explore the speculative truth of the proletariat. This emerges from a rethinking of Marx's concept of the proletariat, which encompasses four fundamental dimensions: psyche, existence, subject, and politics. The conclusion of this book, drawing on the main arguments derived from Chapters 2–6, illustrates the Lacanian formula of proletariat discourse through the diagram (see Figure 8.1).

In the upper left corner of the diagram, the psyche of the proletariat is illustrated. At point S_1, this psyche reflects a realm of thought shaped by social conditions, leading to a lack of a unified identity regarding the proletariat's psyche. Following Hegel's dialectic method, the psyche represents a self-divided entity, which indicates an internal conflict within the proletariat itself. In contrast to the unified definitions presented by psychology, interpreting the proletariat's psyche from a psychoanalytic perspective reveals it to be fragmented and containing undefinable characteristics – similar to a montage. The psyche of the proletariat is shaped by the material conditions of capitalism and does not arise solely from instinct and emotion. Therefore, it can be characterized as materialistic rather than idealistic. In this context, it is important to note that the proletariat's psyche

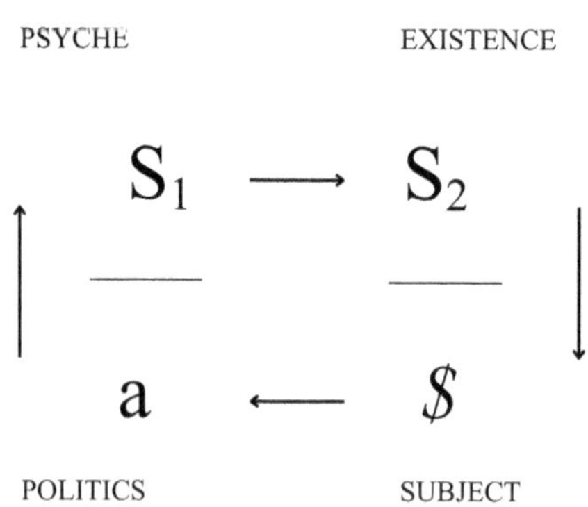

Figure 8.1 Proletariat discourse formula.

Source: Photo by the author

differs from Marx's concept of the proletariat's consciousness, which he defines as class consciousness intertwined with class struggle and antagonism.

In contrast to a positive belief in class consciousness, the psyche can express itself through a form of hysteric. In this context, the proletariat serves as a specter of communism that haunts capitalism, which can lead to a form of aphasia. This suggests that the communist vision held by the proletariat may extend beyond Marx's own imagination of communism and even stand in opposition to Marx's vision of a Kantian utopia. Additionally, the psyche may manifest as alienation, where the proletariat is consumed by capitalism – this represents a lethal form of alienation. Simultaneously, the proletariat strives to oppose this condition, resulting in what can be viewed as a celebrated form of alienation. However, this lethal alienation can create a binding force that disturbs and prevents the proletariat from achieving true separation from capitalism.

The psyche is also linked to enjoyment, which is not merely about pleasure or self-gratification. Instead, the enjoyment of the proletariat reflects moral transgressions, such as those imposed by religious doctrines and moral commandments. Within this framework, the psyche of the proletariat engages in repeated acts of violation across various forms of enjoyment: masochistic enjoyment (the passion for working in the repressive highly reputed companies), sadistic enjoyment (bullying fellow proletariat colleagues), and narcissistic enjoyment (achieving success within the capitalist world by all means necessary). These forms of enjoyment serve not only to fulfill their desires but also to ensure their survival within capitalism, thereby enabling the continuity of the capitalist system itself.

Furthermore, the psyche of the proletariat is intertwined with anxiety, stemming from their awareness of the presence of the object. This anxiety suggests that the proletariat may consent to exist as a source of surplus-value as a coping mechanism, which ultimately undermines their ability to resist capitalism. The triad of trauma – Real-Trauma, Imaginary-Trauma, and Symbolic-Trauma – affects the psyche of the proletariat. Those experiencing Real-Trauma understand the need to oppose capitalism but may struggle to achieve revolutionary change. This can lead to a regression into Imaginary-Trauma (feeling that solidarity is unattainable) and Symbolic-Trauma (viewing politics as merely identity politics), complicating their path to action. Ultimately, this dialectical psychoanalytical condition suggests that traditional Marxism oversimplifies the complexities of proletariat consciousness, believing that merely achieving class consciousness will instantly lead to political revolution.

The upper right corner represents existence. At point S_2, existence refers to the relationship between proletariat and capitalism. Proletariat exists in capitalism; in other words, capitalism forms intersubjectivity with the proletariat. However, this intersubjectivity, or smooth correlation, between the proletariat and capitalism seems to misrepresent the existence of the proletariat. Instead of this intersubjectivity, the proletariat rather *ex-sists* – denoting a negation of or separation from the surrounding being. This separation means realizing the symptom that capitalism imposes on the lives of the proletariat. Hence, it is impossible for them to *ex-sist* without interpreting the capitalist world, its dominance, and various forms of exploitation as a priori. Thus, it can be insisted that the task of philosophy is to interpret the world – understanding the tension between the proletariat and capitalism – before thinking about changing it.

Interpreting capitalism does not imply that it can be changed without experiencing any recessions. The assertion that philosophy's role is to change the world is an optimistic one. In fact, philosophy serves to raise caution and to explain why attempts to change the world based solely on beliefs in solidarity and a united proletariat consistently fail and are nearly impossible. *Ex-sistence* beyond capitalism does not entail either defining a radical identity for the proletariat or avoiding confrontations with reality in a communist society. In cases of a hysterical proletariat, a new communist leader may not be repressive but may struggle to govern effectively due to the proletariat's tendency to obscure the truth from those in power. Unlike Marx's negative view of alienation, the *ex-sistence* of the proletariat involves embracing alienation: it means acknowledging the loss of the old social structures and foundations in order to pave the way for a new way of life that lacks traditional grounding. This peculiar way of life compels proletariats to seek and rediscover a sense of home and suggests an alternative way of living and envisioning the future after capitalism that does not necessarily align with Marx's communist ideal.

The *ex-sistence* of the proletariat is likely hindered by three psychoanalytic dimensions of enjoyment – masochistic, sadistic, and narcissistic – which are intertwined with their self-enjoyment experiences and play an essential role in perpetuating capitalism. Achieving *ex-sistence* is further complicated by intersubjectivity, which can manifest as surplus-value; this serves as a mechanism through which the proletariat seeks to alleviate anxiety and prevent anxiety attacks. Despite the intertwining of *ex-sistence* with dialectical materialism and a distancing from capitalist trauma, it is the notion of communist fantasy that drives both the proletariat and traditional Marxism to confront the Real within the realm of communism, until communism itself remains subject to the laws of dialectics.

The lower right corner represents the concept of the subject. Regarding the barred subject or $, the term "subject" refers to Marx's definition of the proletariat, which emphasizes the proletariat as the labor force that exchanges their work for wages, as well as a subject of resistance to capitalism. It is important to note that Marx's view of the proletariat lacks psychoanalytic insight. His understanding is rooted in economic theory, particularly concerning the connection between the proletariat and surplus-value, framing the proletariat as both a subject of resistance against the existing capitalist system and its superstructure. This perspective results in a limited understanding of the subject. Psychoanalysis plays a crucial role in reexamining Marx's work, helping to broaden the understanding of the proletariat not only as wage laborers but also as subjects of resistance – political agents committed to abolishing capitalism. This perspective also allows for a critical evaluation of the limitations and potential improvements regarding Marx's concept of the proletariat. By employing Lacanian psychoanalysis to emphasize the proletariat's role as a political agency opposing capitalism, it is important to proceed with caution. Psychoanalysis should be seen as a warning to Marxism rather than as a seamless partnership in an ambitious political project.

Concerning the hysterical proletariat, it seems that this form of proletariat subject often resists compromise and compliance with communist doctrine. Deep down, the proletariat embodies a true master who, despite lacking a formal political position, harbors a profound desire that resembles a mystical yearning, capable of shaking and disrupting the entire communist framework. The phallic authoritarian regime known as the dictatorship of the proletariat still grapples with an ontological inconsistency: it is likely that the idea of permanent revolution will eventually fade, not due to capitalism but because of the proletariat themselves. With respect to the contradictory principles at play in the unconscious, it appears that this unconscious operates in a cyclical manner, functioning like a Mobius strip. This could motivate the proletariat, as a resistant subject, to strive for a world beyond capitalism. However, according to the laws of dialectics, the same mechanism of the unconscious may also hinder the proletariat, causing them to slow their progress as a resistant subject and ultimately conform to capitalism, which promises the pleasure principle. This compliance can become a significant obstacle to the proletariat's revolutionary aspirations.

The development of the proletariat into a being of divine enjoyment suggests that divinity still plays a crucial role in shaping the subjectivity of the proletariat. This concept of a non-Christian God can serve as an opium of the proletariat, leading them to believe that they themselves are divine. However, Marx overlooks this belief in divine enjoyment when considering the proletariat as a potential force of resistance against capitalism. Divine enjoyment can diminish due to three modes of self-enjoyment – masochism, sadism, and narcissism – which may shift the proletariat's focus from revolutionary passion back to sustaining capitalism. One important aspect that Marx tends to miss is that the proletariat can be interpreted psychoanalytically as a source of anxiety. First, the proletariat subject embodies action (*passage à l'acte*), facing significant social repercussions until they reach a breaking point, which can lead to depression and withdrawal. Second, resilient proletariat subjects engage in action (acting-out), transforming their ignorance into certainty amidst adversity from other members of society. They refuse to leave the stage and consistently return to it. Ultimately, from the perspective of Lacanian trauma theory, the proletariat can be viewed as a post-traumatic subject – one that is determined to detach itself from the symbolic order and embrace danger. At this critical juncture between the old and the new world, this post-traumatic proletariat must weigh the option of whether to pursue a revolutionary path or to remain confined by the material conditions imposed by capitalism.

The lower left corner represents the politics of the proletariat, a space where the future of society after capitalism remains an object of desire. This political stance does not align with the Lacanian Left, postcolonial politics, radical democracy, or identity politics. While it shares the fundamental principle of emancipation with the Lacanian-Marxist movement – specifically, an anti-capitalist agenda – it requires careful critical examination. One can conceptualize the proletariat as a sublime hysteric, politically antagonistic to the neoliberal university and the unlimited surplus crises of global capitalism. However, this characterization must be approached with caution. The paradoxical nature of the unconscious, as articulated through Lacan's concept of *Spaltung* (or splitting), suggests that there is no guarantee the proletariat, seen as sublime hysterics, will consistently engage in revolutionary actions. Instead, they could disrupt the revolution or undermine the communist vision from within. Furthermore, the proletariat can embrace the notion of divine violence, positioning themselves not just as agents of divine enjoyment but as embodiments of a divine force in their struggle for revolutionary change. Yet, there is no assurance that their engagement with divine enjoyment will remain stable. They may very well revert to forms of masochistic, sadistic, or narcissistic enjoyment, oscillating between cooperation with capitalism and their pursuit of divine enjoyment and violence in resisting it – much like the movement of a Mobius strip.

There exists the presence of a vision for the future called degrowth communism, proposed by a new Marxist figure. This concept is distinctly different from identity politics, postcolonialism, and the Lacanian Left. This vision may represent an object of desire that contrasts with the proletariat's expectations because the proletariat may envision a communist world or an alternative to capitalism, not necessarily aligned with this predefined image. While it is essential for the politics of the proletariat to maintain a critique of capitalism, it is also possible that alternative political movements, such as postcolonial identity politics and radical democracy, can distract the proletariat from this universalism. Instead of abolishing capitalism, they may divert attention toward other paths of emancipation. At this moment, it might be too late to address the question: do proletariats have the courage not to stray from this pursuit of progress, an abolition of capitalism as universalism, and to develop an ontological consistency in solidarity? Their subjectivities must contend with these internal dynamics of dialectics. The solidarity of the proletariat is highly questionable due to differences in race, language, sexuality, and nationality. While calling for global proletariat solidarity is necessary, it often appears to be an illusion. If the call for solidarity among the proletariat worldwide is merely a fantasy, then the future after capitalism can be represented as *objet a*: the object of desire that lies beyond the confines of capitalism. This object is present yet often just out of reach – it serves as a sticking point in the Marxist symbolic representation of the envisioned future after capitalism.

Ultimately, the thesis of proletariat discourse emphasizes the need for a critical and comprehensive reappraisal and rethinking of Marxism, particularly regarding the concept of the proletariat. It highlights a significant disparity between Lacanian psychoanalysis and Marxism, rather than suggesting a direct homology. This highlights the differences between the condition of the proletariat in Marx's era and that of the present time. Not only does it encourage new thinking about the proletariat as a political agency but also hopes that this critical reinterpretation of Marxism through a Lacanian psychoanalytic lens will enhance Marxism and contribute to the broader intellectual development of Marxist philosophy.

Index

For Product Safety Concerns and Information please contact our EU representative GPSR@taylorandfrancis.com Taylor & Francis Verlag GmbH, Kaufingerstraße 24, 80331 München, Germany

Batch number: 10482770

Printed by Printforce, the Netherlands